GW00696677

Homoeopathy

Homoeopathy

A critical appraisal

Editors

Edzard Ernst MD, PhD, FRCP (Edin)
Director, Department of Complementary Medicine,
Postgraduate Medical School, University of Exeter, UK

Eckhart G. Hahn MD, FACP
Director, Department of Medicine I, University of Erlangen,
Germany

Assistant Editors

Benno Brinkhaus MD
Acting Head, Division of Complementary Medicine I,
University of Erlangen, Germany

Christian Hentschel MD
Director, Modellklinik Naturheilkunde für
Nordrhein-Westfalen, Germany

Gernot Schindler
Research Associate, Division of Complementary Medicine,
Department of Medicine I, University of Erlangen, Germany

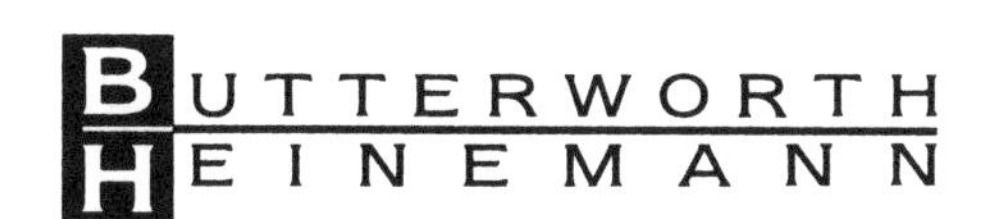

Butterworth-Heinemann
Linacre House, Jordan Hill, Oxford OX2 8DP
225 Wildwood Avenue, Woburn, MA 01801-2041
A division of Reed Educational and Professional Publishing Ltd

A member of the Reed Elsevier plc group

OXFORD BOSTON JOHANNESBURG
MELBOURNE NEW DELHI SINGAPORE

First published 1998

British Library Cataloguing in Publication Data
A catalogue record for this book is available from the British Library

Library of Congress Cataloguing in Publication Data
A catalogue record for this book is available from the Library of Congress

ISBN 0 7506 3564 9

Typeset by Latimer Trend & Company Ltd, Plymouth
Printed and bound in Great Britain by Biddles Ltd, Guildford and King's Lynn

Contents

Part IV: Experimental Studies

Part V: Socioeconomic Aspects

Contributors

Gerassimos S. Anagnostatos National Center for Scientific Research, 'Demokritos', Institute of Nuclear Physics, Aghia Paraskevi, Attiki, Greece

Benno Brinkhaus Head of Research Group for Traditional and Complementary Medicine, Department of Medicine I, Friedrich-Alexander University Erlangen-Nuremberg, Erlangen, Germany

Nicola Clausius Projekt 'Münchener Modell', Ludwig-Maximilians-Universität München, Germany

Flávio Dantas Professor of Medical Ethics and Homoeopathy, Department of Clinical Medicine, Federal University of Uberlândia (Brazil) and Visiting Research Fellow (1995–96), The Royal London Homoeopathic Hospital NHS Trust, London, UK

Joachim H. Dittmann Institut für Physiologische Chemie, Tierärztliche Hochschule Hannover, Hannover, Germany

Florian Eitel Theoretische Chirurgie, Chirurgische Klinik und Poliklinik Innestadt, Ludwig-Maximilians-Universität, München, Germany

John M. English Homoeopathic Medical Research Council, Salisbury, UK

Edzard Ernst Director, Department of Complementary Medicine, Postgraduate Medical School, University of Exeter, Exeter, Devon, UK

Peter Fisher Director of Research, The Royal London Homoeopathic Hospital NHS Trust, London, UK

Adrian Furnham Department of Psychology, University College London, London, UK

Wilhelm Gaus Department of Biometry and Medical Documentation, University of Ulm, Ulm, Germany

Eckhart G. Hahn Professor, Director of Medical Department I, Friedrich-Alexander University Erlangen-Nuremberg, Germany

Günther Harisch Institut für Physiologische Chemie, Tierärztliche Hochschule Hannover, Hannover, Germany

Larry V. Hedges Department of Education, The University of Chicago, Chicago, Illinois, USA, UK

Christian Hentschel Director, Blankenstein Hospital, Department of Complementary Medicine, Hattingen, Germany

Alexandra Jansen Research Group for Traditional and Complementary Medicine, Department of Medicine I, Friedrich-Alexander University Erlangen-Nuremberg, Erlangen, Germany

Wayne B. Jonas Director, Office of Alternative Medicine, National Institutes of Health, Bethesda, Maryland, USA

Ralf Kohnen Professor, Director, Institute of Psychology II, Friedrich-Alexander University Erlangen-Nuremberg, Germany

Martina Kron Department of Biometry and Medical Documentation, University of Ulm, Ulm, Germany

Walter Lehmacher Institut für Medizinische Statistik, Informatik und Epidemiologie, Universität zu Köln, Germany

Klaus Linde 'Münchener Modell', Centre for Complementary Medicine Research, Technical University, Ludwig-Maximilians-Universität München, Germany

Martin Lindner Research Group for Traditional and Complementary Medicine, Department of Medicine I, Friedrich-Alexander University Erlangen-Nuremberg, Erlangen, Germany

Dieter Melchart 'Münchener Modell', Centre for Complementary Medicine Research, Technical University, Ludwig-Maximilians-Universität München, Germany

Polykarpos Pissis National Technical University of Athens, Physics Department, Polytechneiopolis, Zografou, Athens, Greece

Fritz-Albert Popp Visiting Professr (mult.), International Institute of Biophysics, Raketenstation, Neuss, Germany

Gilbert Ramirez Department of Public Health and Preventive Medicine, University of North Texas Health Science Center, Fort Worth, Texas, USA

David Reilly Consultant Physician, Glasgow Homoeopathic Hospital, Glasgow. Also Honorary Senior Lecturer, University Department of Medicine, The University of Glasgow, UK

Gernot Schindler Research Group for Traditional and Complementary Medicine, Department of Medicine I, Friedrich-Alexander University Erlangen-Nuremberg, Erlangen, Germany

Maria Soutzidou Kapodistrian University of Athens, Physical Chemistry Laboratory, Panepistimiopolis, Athens, Greece

Roeland van Wijk Department of Molecular Cell Biology, Faculty of Biology, Utrecht University, Utrecht, The Netherlands

Kyriakos Viras Kapodistrian University of Athens, Physical Chemistry Laboratory, Panepistimiopolis, Athens, Greece

Harald Walach Universität Freiburg, Psychologisches Institut, Abtg. Rehabilitationspsychologie, Freiburg, Germany

Adrian White Research Fellow, Department of Complementary Medicine, Postgraduate Medical School, University of Exeter, UK

Fred A. C. Wiegant Department of Molecular Cell Biology, Faculty of Biology, Utrecht University, Utrecht, The Netherlands

Frank Wieland Homoeopathic physician, Freiburg, Germany

Introduction

It is 200 years since the German physician Samuel Hahnemann (1755–1843) discovered (or was thought to have discovered) homoeopathy. In 1796 he noticed during experiments on himself that, after taking the malaria remedy quinine, he experienced symptoms similar to those of patients with malaria. Such tests, later termed 'provings' (German: Arzneimittelprüfungen), were repeated on himself, his family and friends and the basic principle was apparently confirmed. Hahnemann drew the conclusion that, if a compound caused symptoms in healthy volunteers, it should then also serve as a remedy for patients who suffer from such symptoms. This hypothesis was apparently confirmed in the therapeutic setting. The 'similia similibus curentur' principle was born.

In the course of his experiments, Hahnemann also noted that diluting and vigorously shaking his remedies, a process later termed 'potentization', rendered the remedy no less active but more potent in terms of clinical response. This was apparently true even for dilutions so high that they were unlikely to contain a single molecule of the original material (the mother tincture). This led Hahnemann to believe that water could display some sort of memory, and that biological activity could be displayed in the absence of the original molecule linked with this activity. The two basic axioms of homoeopathy (like cures like and memory of water) have survived to the present day even though they seem to fly in the face of science.

The undeniable initial success of homoeopathy has to be seen against its historical background. In Hahnemann's days, scientific medicine was still well in its infancy. The therapeutic repertoire was limited, mostly ineffective and often outright hazardous, e.g. blood-letting, purging or prescribing drugs containing poisons like mercury. By contrast homoeopathy, if nothing else, was devoid of serious adverse effects. It is also likely that it produced powerful placebo effects. Thus it took Europe and the USA by storm. At the turn of the century in the USA, 8 per cent of all medical practitioners were homoeopaths, there were 20 homoeopathic colleges, approximately 130 homoeopathic hospitals and 31 homoeopathic medical journals (Ernst and Kaptchuk, 1996).

But even in these early days, criticism from mainstream medicine was intense. The rationale of homoeopathy was denied and therapeutic successes were attributed purely to placebo effects – a situation that has hardly changed since. Homoeopathy therefore remains a challenging and controversial subject. Nevertheless, today it is once again widely accepted among patients. The market for homoeopathic remedies in 1995 was considerable (Germany $528m, France $503m, Netherlands $127m, UK $30m, and the annual predicted growth rate is 15–20 per cent for the next five years (Fasihi, 1996).

Several honest attempts have been made to arrive at the truth with respect to homoeopathy (e.g. Ernst and Kaptchuk, 1996; Kleijnen *et al.*, 1991). However, many discussions on the subject are loaded with prejudice, self-interest and emotion; certainly few books that scrutinize homoeopathy in an objective way exist.

The aim of this volume is to assemble the evidence for or against homoeopathy in a fair and balanced manner. The book brings together the facts regarding three aspects of homoeopathy: clinical evidence; basic research and the socioeconomic relevance of this form of medicine. It is our hope that this volume will be a valuable contribution to the ongoing discussion that has fascinated physicians, scientists and the public for two centuries.

References

Ernst, E. and Kaptchuk, T.J. (1996) Homoeopathy revisited. *Arch. Int. Med.*, **156**, 2162–4.

Fasihi, A. (1996) *Complementary Medicine*, Vol. I. FT Pharmaceuticals and Healthcare Publications, London.

Kleijnen, J., Knipschild, P. and ter Riet, G. (1991) Clinical trials of homoeopathy. *Br. Med. J.*, **302**, 316–32.

Part I

Methodology

Chapter 1

Methodological principles in clinical trials

Walter Lehmacher

Introduction

It is commonly accepted nowadays in the medical research area, that the efficacy of a medical treatment has to be shown by a Randomized Controlled Clinical Trial (RCCT). This is generally accepted as a gold standard from researchers by general scientific principles as well as requested from official agencies by formal guidelines and instructions. Not only new medical treatments have to be evaluated; even well-known and established treatments have to be re-evaluated by well conducted clinical studies.

In homoeopathy there are now two lines of argument. One side says the 200-year-old tradition of homoeopathy and the daily observations of practitioners give enough evidence of its efficacy, and therefore no controlled clinical trials are necessary. Further arguments against RCCTs are that the individualistic approach of homoeopathy makes systematic trials impossible. The other side argues that, even in homoeopathy, RCCTs are possible and therefore necessary, and systematic empirical research based on RCCTs is essential.

Below, the general methodology of modern clinical research is briefly summarized on pp. 4–6. In the next section, the application of these general principles to homoeopathy is described. Conclusions and discussions of these results are then given.

General principles of clinical research

In clinical research, the efficacy of a treatment A cannot be assessed purely by the observation of a single group of patients treated with A, because the natural course of the disease and other co-factors can be the reason for the improvement of the state of the treated patients. Because a potential treatment effect can generally be confounded with other effects, no method of observation and analysis can clearly separate these mixtures of effects.

That is why a control group is necessary. The *comparison* of the treatment A group with the *control* group B gives evidence of a treatment *difference* between A and B and consequently of a treatment *effect* of A. A second choice of control groups would be historical controls. Of course, retrospective or historic controls can be helpful for an insight into a treatment effect, but

Table 1.1 Essentials of a controlled clinical trial

Concurrent controls
- –placebo
- –standard
- –both, or multiple controls

Blinding
- –patients
- –investigators
- –both (double-blinded)

Randomization
- –random assignment of therapies

the comparison with external controls can generally be biased by several co-factors like time trends or by other unknown study specific differences like poorer prognosis of historic controls, too. Unplanned observational studies give no completely convincing contribution for the assessment of efficacy. Therefore, a concurrent *within*-study control is required.

Another aspect of avoiding bias is the application of the principle of *blinding* methods, i.e. of masking the patients and the observers.

A further requirement of reducing bias is *randomization* in order to make sure that the assignment of treatments to patients is free from other, conscious or unconscious, influences and not confounded by other factors. The technique of randomization is nowadays refined for special application, e.g. blocking by prognostic factors.

An additional requirement is that the results of a well planned and conducted trial have to be evaluated by *statistical* methods. This respects the fact that the reactions of the included patients have a biological variability, and only a proper statistical analysis can separate random effects and systematic treatment effects. Statistical methods are also applied in the planning of a trial, e.g. for calculating an adequate sample size.

A first historical example, which respects some of these requirements, is the well-known scorbut experiment of Lind in the year 1747; citations and references are given in Pocock (1983). Further historical examples can be found in Pocock, too.

In Germany, Martini (1932, 1938, 1953, 1968) formulated these methodological requirements of systematic clinical research. He argued that the introduction of therapeutical experiments in medicine has a similar impact as Galilei's foundation of experimental physics.

In the early 1950s, Hill (1951) developed the application and methodology of RCCTs in Great Britain and several large and multi-centre trials were conducted in the USA.

The hierarchy of the strength of evidence concerning the efficacy of a treatment is summarized in Table 1.2 (Green and Byar, 1984). There are multiple potential sources of systematic bias in observational studies. Pitfalls in the unplanned analysis of observational data are well-known in the epidemiological and clinical literature. Only RCCTs can avoid bias in treatment assignment and are most suitable to give empirical evidence as to which of several treatments is the best. Nowadays it is generally accepted

Table 1.2 Hierarchy of strength of evidence concerning efficacy of treatment

Green and Byar, 1984:
1.–Anecdotal case reports
2.–Case series without controls
3.–Series with literature controls
4.–Analyses using computer databases
5.–Case-control observational studies
6.–Series based on historical control groups
7.–Simple randomized controlled clinical trials
8.–Confirmed randomized control clinical trials (including meta-analysis)
Olkin, 1995:
9.–Meta-analysis with original data

by the medical scientific community that a well planned, conducted and analysed RCCT is the principal method for obtaining reliable evaluation of a medical treatment on patients. This is also reflected in the regulations of publication policies of highly respected journals or by the requirements of the national drug administrations. Even complementary therapies have to be evaluated according to these principles; see Ernst and Resch, 1996. Realistic alternatives for proving causality of the treatment and the effect do not exist.

Because a single trial has a certain chance for a false positive result, *reproducibility* is required in the sense that independent replications of successful trials are needed for confirmation. This was clearly demanded since the 1980s; see Green and Byar, 1984, and Table 1.2. In general, the replications should be done preferably by other research groups. The combination of the trials' result can be analysed by meta-analyses; see Olkin, 1995.

The basic principles mentioned above are refined for special applications: e.g. there are special study types like more treatment comparisons, factorial designs for the evaluation of drug combinations, parallel groups or cross-over designs, sequential plans, multi-centre trials, etc. Several biostatistical methods have been developed or adapted for special problems like survival analysis, analysis of repeated measures or multiple endpoints.

In the two last decades, the *quality* of the studies was raised by the demand for a clear *a priori* formulation of all details in the study protocol like focusing on carefully chosen primary endpoints as suitable outcome measures, defining the primary study population with precise inclusion and exclusion criteria, and prespecified statistical analysis methods. All steps of randomization, blinding, data generation and data management have to be accurately planned, conducted and documented in order to check-up all parts of a trial. The modern requirements of good clinical (research) practice (GCP) are collected in textbooks (e.g. Spriet and Dupin-Spriet, 1992), in scientific guidelines (e.g. The Standards of Reporting Trials Group, 1994), and even in official requirements (e.g. EC-CPMP, 1995).

A recent initiative is the Cochrane Collaboration, where a systematic overview of *all* studies concerning a special treatment is tried. In order to avoid the publication bias, which is induced by an over-reporting of successful studies, all planned studies are registered. Later on, *all* study results are collected, even the results of negative and non-published trials, and systematically analysed with meta-analyses (Chalmers and Altman, 1995).

Application in homoeopathy

In homoeopathy, well conducted RCCTs are possible. After an initial assessment, if patients with a certain disease and indication are suitable for the specific homoeopathic therapy under consideration, the patients are included in the trial and then randomized. A double-blinded application of the homoeopathic drug or control drug can be organized in the usual way. The feasibility of RCCTs in homoeopathy is demonstrated by several well conducted trials; examples can be found in the review articles of Hill and Doyon (1990) and Kleijnen *et al.* (1991) and in recent studies like Wiesenauer and Gaus (1993) or Gaus (1994).

The specific problems in homoeopathy are not fundamentally larger than in some other fields of medicine. For example, if blinding in surgery is a problem, a second doctor makes the assessments of the success of the surgical intervention. Or if individual dose finding and individual adaptation of drugs in psychiatry is a problem, the change or adaptation of the verum drugs can be organized respecting double blinding. If, in oncology, not only two drugs but several therapeutic strategies are to be compared, special central randomization procedures can be applied in order to make sure that randomization is well conducted even in unblinded trials. In several fields of medical research, the general methodological issues of RCCTs are adapted to specific solutions, e.g. with external assessments, or more complicated study types like more armed trials, crossover trials (Lehmacher, 1991) or change-of-treatment trials (Ernst and Resch, 1995).

Indeed, several homoeopathic trials respecting the methods of RCCTs are conducted. About 200 RCCTs of homoeopathy have been published. The majority of these studies are 'positive' in the sense that the homoeopathic drugs under consideration show a better effect than the concurrent placebos. But a large proportion of these positive studies have major methodological problems concerning clinical aspects or they lack clear statistical evidence.

The fact that the majority of published studies are positive is no proof of the efficacy of homoeopathy. It is well-known that research groups in the academic field, as well as drug companies, are enthusiastic in publishing their positive results. But in most cases a negative result is deemed to be not scientifically important or not commercially helpful. Therefore negative results are very often not published. The publication policy of journals also favours positive results, because positive trials give an evidence for a positive effect, where negative trials give no clear interpretation, because the effect can be missing or the study has methodological deficiencies, e.g. wrong endpoints are chosen or the sample sizes are too small. The author's own experience from statistical consulting in the academic and industrial area confirms this behaviour. Thus a selection of positive studies in the sense of overreporting or overpublishing them is a fact in all areas of medical research. This well-known phenomenon is called *publication bias*. The proportion of positive studies among the published studies in homoeopathy can be explained fairly by a publication bias.

This problem is familiar in many other fields of therapeutic research. A solution is that positive studies have to be repeated, and the independent replications of the main results are a necessary requisite of a proof of efficacy. The only meta-analysis of homoeopathic studies seems to be the one of Reilly *et al.* (1994). Further replications of successful homoeopathic studies and their combinations by meta-analyses seem to be missing.

Hill and Doyon (1990) conclude in their overview of homoeopathic RCCTs, that '. . . the results do not provide acceptable evidence that homoeopathic treatments are effective'.

Kleijnen, Knipschild and ter Riet (1991) conclude: 'At the moment the evidence of clinical trials is positive but not sufficient to draw definitive conclusions because most trials are of low methodological quality and because of the unknown role of publication bias. This indicates that there is a legitimate case for further evaluation of homoeopathy, but only by means of well performed trials.'

All newer presentations of overviews of homoeopathic trials show a large proportion of positive studies among the studies included in the review (Linde and Melchart, 1996). But none of them show replication of positive studies; publication bias alone can explain the percentage of positive studies. Because there is no systematic registration of all planned and finished homoeopathic studies, a complete overview and analysis of positive *and* negative studies is not possible.

Conclusions and discussion

In the author's view there is a certain amount of positive evidence of efficacy of homoeopathic drugs, but:

- many 'positive' studies have methodological problems and the interpretation of their results gives no clear evidence;
- a consistent confirmation of study results by independent replications is needed;
- the proportion of positive studies can be explained by publication bias;
- further RCCTs are necessary, especially the independent replication of positive studies.

RCCTs are necessary in clinical research for methodological reasons. They are feasible in homoeopathy, and therefore they are necessary. Homoeopathic doctors should accept this fact, and not discuss why and how to avoid RCCTs. At present the results of RCCTs are not convincing. Further RCCTs are urgently needed in homoeopathy, in order to confirm or to disprove it. A systematic documentation of all planned and finished trials has to be organized according to the initiative of the Cochrane Collaboration. The chance of realization of these missing last steps is large and easy to perform.

Homoeopathy has to face this challenge, or it disappears. The Oracle of Delphi was accepted for 1000 years, the method of blood-letting was over-emphasized for 500 years, and the 200-year tradition of homoeopathy is no final proof of its efficacy.

References

Chalmers, I. and Altmann, D.G. (eds), (1995) *Systematic Reviews.* BMJ Publishing Group, London.

EC-CPMP (1995) Biostatistical Methodology in Clinical Trials in Applications for Marketing Authorization for Medicinal Products. *Stat. Med.*, **14**, 1659–82.

Ernst, E. and Resch, K.L. (1995) The 'Optional Cross-Over Design' for Randomized Controlled Trials. *Fundam. Clin. Pharmacol.*, **9**, 508–11.

Ernst, E. and Resch, K.L. (1996) Evaluating Specific Effectiveness of Complementary Therapies – A Position Paper. (Part One: Methodological Aspects). *Forsch. Komplementärmed.*, **3**, 35–8.

Gaus, W. (1994) Biometrischer Auswertungsbericht der Studie 'Die Wirksamkeit der klassischen homöopathischen Therapie bei chronischen Kopfschmerzen'. Department Biometry, Medical School, University Ulm, unpublished.

Green, S.B. and Byar, D.P. (1984) Using Observational Data from Registries to Compare Treatments: The Fallacy of Omnimetrics. *Stat. Med.*, **3**, 361–70.

Hill, A.B. (1951) The Clinical Trial. *Brit. Med. Bull.*, **7**, 278–82.

Hill, C. and Doyon, F. (1990) Review of Randomized Trials of Homoeopathy. *Rev. Epidém. et Santé Public.*, **38**, 138–47.

Kleijnen, J., Knipschild, P. and ter Riet, G. (1991) Clinical Trials of Homoeopathy. *Brit. Med. J.*, **302**, 316–23.

Lehmacher, W. (1991) Analysis of the Cross-Over Design in the Presence of Residual Effects. *Stat. Med.*, **10**, 891–9.

Linde, K. and Melchart, D. (1996) Der Wirksamkeitsnachweis der Homöopathie – eine unendliche Geschichte? *Dt. Apothekerzeitung*, **136**, 2679–84.

Martini, P. (1932, 1938, 1953, 1968) *Methodenlehre der therapeutisch-klinischen Forschung.* Springer, Heidelberg.

Olkin, I. (1995) Meta-Analysis: Reconciling the Results of Independent Studies. *Stat. Med.*, **14**, 457–72.

Pocock, S.J. (1983) *Clinical Trials.* Wiley, New York.

Reilly, D., Taylor, M.A., Beattle, N.G.M., Campbell, J.H., McSharry, C., Aitchison, T.C., Carter, R. and Stevenson, R.D. (1994) Is Evidence for Homoeopathy Reproducible? *Lancet*, **344**, 1601–6.

Spriet, A. and Dupin-Spriet, T. (1992) *Good Practice of Clinical Drug Trials.* Karger, Basel.

The Standards of Reporting Trials Group (1994) A Proposal for Structured Reporting of Randomized Controlled Clinical Trials. *J. Am. Med. Assoc.*, **272**, 1926–31.

Wiesenauer, M. and Gaus, W. (1993) Wirksamkeitsnachweis eines Homöopathikums bei chronischer Polyarthritis. *Akt. Rheumatol.*, **16**, 1–9.

Chapter 2

Guidelines on methodology of clinical research in homoeopathy

Martina Kron, John M. English and Wilhelm Gaus

Acknowledgement

The European Commission sponsored the Homoeopathic Medicine Research Group chaired by Georges Fülgraff (Berlin). Jean Pierre Boissel (Lyon), Jacques Dangoumau (Bordeaux), John M. English (Salisbury), Wilhelm Gaus, co-ordinator (Ulm), Martina Kron (Ulm), Elisabeth S.M. deLange-deKlerk (Amsterdam), David Reilly (Glasgow) and Frank Wieland (Freiburg) participated in the research methodology subgroup. These guidelines on methodology of clinical research in homoeopathy are a slightly modified result of the work of this subgroup. The report of the entire group including a dictionary of homoeopathic terms is available from the European Commission, Directorate General XII, Science, Research and Development, Life Sciences and Technologies, Medical Research, Rue de la Loi 200, B-1049 Brussels.

Methodological problems of clinical research specific to homoeopathy

In view of the peculiarities of homoeopathy, designing clinical studies is difficult. Special requirements for differing homoeopathic strategies may lead to the following methodological problems when planning and designing clinical studies. Some problems are specific to certain strategies, some are similar to those in other unconventional therapies (Gaus and Högel, 1995; Righetti, 1988). As homoeopathic pathological prescribing is similar to conventional medicine, it has fewer particular problems than classical homoeopathy.

Individualized therapy

Classical homoeopathic treatment is highly individualized. The choice of the remedy depends not only on anamnesis, symptoms and disease but also on aetiology, lifestyle, constitution, personality and many other issues.

Some circumstances, which include other modalities such as special nutrition or psychotherapeutical care, have to be accounted for which might be difficult under study conditions, especially because they have to be standardized. Ideally, the homoeopathic remedy should be the only difference, either as the sole treatment, or the sole addition to a mandatory standardized conventional regime.

There are elements of homoeopathic treatment apart from application of medicines which are essentials of homoeopathic treatment, especially in classical homoeopathy. Important factors are the attention to emotions and the patient's personal problems, psychological support and explanation of symptoms. Treatments are difficult to standardize because of differences between homoeopathic healers and schools.

Management of therapeutic failure

In any clinical trial there will be some patients who fail to respond to the treatment they receive. In a homoeopathic clinical trial, this might be due to:

- being in the placebo section of the trial;
- being in the verum section, but they received the wrong remedy;
- being in the verum section, but they received the right remedy, in the wrong potency;
- being in the verum section, but they received the right remedy, in the right potency, but there were external factors acting against its action (those known in homoeopathy as 'obstacles to cure'). For example, some patients who continue to drink coffee might fail to respond, whereas others would be unaffected;
- the diagnosis might have been wrong, or another illness might have developed;
- for reasons unknown, the patient might be unable to respond to homoeopathic treatment. Susceptibility is believed to vary.

Depending on the severity of the patient's condition, one of the following courses of action would be necessary:

- in the patient's interest the doctor in charge decides to break the trial code and administers whatever treatment is needed at the point reached;
- the patient decides to leave the trial;
- the failure to respond is not great enough to result in either of the above, so the trial continues. This would apply in the majority of cases.

The possibility of having failed to find the right homoeopathic treatment is one which faces homoeopathic physicians in a way which is quite different from the conventional trial (Walach, 1996) in which the treatment options are predetermined once the diagnosis is made.

In cases where the patient continues in the trial, i.e. the masking of the treatment groups is maintained in spite of poor treatment success, unbiased results of the study can be obtained. Then the homoeopath should presume that the patient received the homoeopathic remedy and should ignore the possibility that it might also have been placebo.

Outcome variables

In general, four different types of outcome variables are recognized:

- outcome variables measuring effects (any observed effect, any biological change in relation to the treatment);
- outcome variables measuring efficacy (improvement of the primary outcome variable);
- outcome variables measuring benefit, i.e. improvement of quality of life, prolongation of lifetime;
- outcome variables measuring patient satisfaction.

The primary goal of homoeopathy is improving health and restoring the feeling of well-being. Homoeopathy considers the patient in his/her entirety, and does not primarily cure symptoms. Healing the disease and amelioration of symptoms is a consequence of improved general health status. Beside quality of life and well-being instruments, other instruments have to be developed to measure quantitatively the whole of what the homoeopath seeks to achieve. New instruments are necessary because treatment success is often assessed indirectly by assessing changes in symptoms. This might be done for example by subjective evaluation of pain or health status, which is often less reliable, less objective and less valid.

Homoeopathic therapy would be preferred to conventional therapy even if it were only equally effective, as far fewer adverse drug reactions are expected.

Initial aggravation

There is the phenomenon known as the homoeopathic aggravation, which is a worsening of symptoms occurring soon after the administration of a remedy, or a reappearance of symptoms associated with a past pathology. Either of these is usually of short duration and not severe. According to clinical experience, such an aggravation has a good prognostic value. This eventuality will have been fully explained to participants, and is therefore unlikely to result in withdrawal from a trial.

Treatment duration

The homoeopathic treatment of chronic illness may take a long time to take effect (Ritter, 1966). The length to follow-up in such situations could be as much as 1–2 years. Long term clinical studies are difficult to organize, expensive and time consuming. Although the effect is measured after a long time, the treatment effect is often only small and small treatment effects need large sample sizes. Moreover, long term therapy with placebo has ethical objections (see under Ethical issues p. 14).

Another drawback is that a long treatment duration may result in many drop-outs, either from lack of response, or because they are better and see no need for further treatment. For drop-outs the study outcome variable cannot be measured, thus drop-outs can bias the study results.

In general cross-over designs are unsuitable for long term therapy, and especially for homoeopathy, because homoeopaths believe that their medicines have a profound and long-lasting effect. Therefore, only parallel group designs are appropriate.

Patients' conviction

The potential placebo effect of homoeopathy might be increased where the patient has a positive view of the subject, or vice-versa. It might be worthwhile to ascertain by questionnaire what each entrant's expectation was, as it is a potential source of bias. The possibility prejudices recruitment either from homoeopaths' own practices or from media advertisement. Even patients recruited from a specialist clinic not directly involved with homoeopathy are likely to produce some bias because they might have negative attitudes towards homoeopathy.

Sometimes only a few patients give informed consent to participate in a randomized masked trial. Some patients might refuse to participate in a clinical trial in which they could be randomized to placebo or conventional therapy, because they are convinced of the efficacy of the homoeopathic remedy. Thus, the patients participating in a study might be a biased sample and the generalizability and applicability of study results is restricted. However, it would be a remarkable progress if for instance the efficacy of homoeopathy could be demonstrated in a convincing way for a certain subgroup of patients.

Therapists' conviction

Some homoeopaths are so convinced of the efficacy of their treatment or so averse to what they see as the distortion of good homoeopathic practice by the constraints of the trial discipline, that they would not agree to participate in such a trial and to randomize their patients to placebo or a conventional treatment.

Patient–therapist relationship

In homoeopathy a special relationship develops between patient and therapist. Case taking will be complicated or sometimes even impossible if the relationship is poor. In this case the likelihood of a successful homoeopathic prescription being identified is prejudiced.

Factors connected with the trial which might tend to affect the consultation include:

- for the doctor, not knowing to which group (verum or placebo) the patient belongs. This will affect follow-up consultations more than the first one;
- for the patient, being in a trial and being videoed, if that is a requirement (if it is, the patient will already have agreed to it).

Placebo and homoeopathic therapy

Homoeopathic history- and case-taking is recognized as having a considerable psychological effect. It may affect the outcome to the extent that even placebo group patients may benefit from the history-taking (see under Necessity of a control group p. 29 for reasons for treatment success under placebo).

The ideal choice of substance used as a placebo is a matter for debate. For instance, it could be the vehicle (alcohol, milk-sugar) potentized without remedy or the plain (unpotentized) vehicle. The members of the Konsensus-Conference of the Karl and Veronica Carstens-Stiftung recommended for reasons of external and internal validity the unpotentized vehicle of the homoeopathic remedy as placebo (e.g. alcohol, a water-alcohol mixture or lactose; Albrecht and Frühwald, 1995). It is imperative that the substance chosen as placebo must be clearly stated in every study protocol.

Therapists' qualification

A study in homoeopathic medicine cannot be conducted by non-homoeopathically oriented therapists. It requires homoeopathically trained physicians of considerable experience. Poor results in some studies are attributable to failure in this respect. A minimum of five years' homoeopathic practice and familiarity with the conditions under investigation have been suggested, and are reasonable requirements. It is in fact desirable that the research team include uncommitted research experts. Centres of recognized reputation for research in the field should be sought wherever possible. They will help both to ensure a high standard of research practice, and give credence to the results. Problems will arise in the attempt to identify eligible study centres and in defining and standardizing the treatment to make results comparable.

Launching studies by practitioners in private practice is complicated by the lack of methodological interest of many practitioners and the personal and financial relationship between patient and physician (the physician does not want to lose his patient). The advantages of studies in an out-patient clinic situation are the possibility of recruiting sufficient patients within a short time if many physicians agree to participate, and the results of such studies are easy to generalize and important for the treatment of chronic diseases in practice.

Homoeopathic physicians come from different schools, have different experiences and therefore select different remedies. However, some or all prescriptions might be (equally) effective.

Ethical issues

There should be sufficient grounds for anticipating a positive clinical effect before a trial is authorized. The evidence for this in the case of homoeopathic studies is often low, as so little research has taken place. Therefore, it is necessary to launch further studies in homoeopathy planned to demonstrate its efficacy. Attention should be paid to the fact that the trial should not cover ground which has already been adequately researched.

Homoeopathic therapy is said to be safe and has usually no serious adverse drug reactions. It therefore meets this ethical requirement.

Some consider it unethical to give a patient placebo for a long time. The length of the trial might thus give rise to ethical objections on this count. Emergency treatment has to be available to all patients under the terms of the trial protocol. In some cases, standard conventional treatment must be continued, the homoeopathy/placebo being added to it.

The protocol must adhere to and state that it adheres to Good Clinical Practice and the Declaration of Helsinki (see also under GCP regulations p. 5). The patient must be allowed to withdraw from the trial at any time. To be informed about the trial, its purpose, its risks and possible outcomes is the right of every patient, who must give consent. The names, positions and addresses of those involved in the trial, and their relevant experience justifying their participation in it, are to appear in the study protocol. The trial protocol should be registered and an intention affirmed to publish regardless of the results.

Scope of clinical research in homoeopathy

Research questions

There are many research questions regarding homoeopathy, to which the answers are of great interest for patients, for homoeopaths and for the scientific community.

Efficacy

Homoeopathy claims to cure by supporting the patient's innate defence mechanisms, and not by the control and suppression of symptoms. The mechanism by which this is achieved, assuming it is, remains unproven. It must be addressed by later research, some of which will depend on laboratory studies which clarify the nature of ultramolecular, succussed dilutions.

The mechanism of action of many conventional drugs is unknown, even though their efficacy has been demonstrated in controlled clinical trials. This approach could also be possible in homoeopathy. Two (or more) groups of patients get different treatments for some time and then the averaged therapeutical success achieved in each group is compared. This approach is purely empirical and does not require any theory how the investigated therapy works in the body.

Maybe research in homoeopathy is more difficult, more complicated than in conventional medicine. However, the practical approach is – to some extent – applicable to any type of medical therapy. The specific methodological problems of clinical research in homoeopathy are given on p. 9, but we are convinced that today's methodology enables us to solve at least some of the problems of clinical research in homoeopathy and addresses some of the research questions described in this Section.

The following examples are questions on efficacy.

- Does homoeopathy cure or significantly alleviate the pathology of a certain disease?
- Are the results of homoeopathy attributable to placebo action?
- Does homoeopathy reduce symptoms caused by a certain disease?
- Does homoeopathy improve the quality of life in patients with a certain disease?
- What global effects are found from homoeopathic treatment of patients?
- Are there differences in efficacy of homoeopathic therapy in daily practice and in a clinical research project?

The patients investigated, their disease(s) and the relevant diagnostic criteria are defined by the inclusion and exclusion criteria of the study protocol. How therapeutic success is expressed – by symptoms, survival time, quality of life or patient's satisfaction – is established in the study protocol by the definition of outcome variables.

Different sections of the community hold different views on the priorities for homoeopathic research. The scientific community currently assumes that the primary research task is to determine whether the response to homoeopathic remedies is larger than a placebo response. The smaller the difference in outcome, the greater the sample size needed for the difference to become significant. Hence, from the methodological point of view it is easier to show efficacy, i.e. a larger difference in outcome, than to show a minor improvement. This strategy attempts to prove the efficacy of homoeopathy first, and then – when efficacy of homoeopathy is widely accepted by the scientific community – proceeds to studies improving and optimizing homoeopathic effectiveness (see also under Efficacy p. 27).

Practicability

Questions on practicability are concerned with practical organization, cost-effectiveness, integration in conventional medicine and qualification in homoeopathy. Within this context questions arise like:

- Which diseases do homoeopaths treat successfully?
- In which diseases is homoeopathic treatment cost-effective?
- What staff and facilities does a homoeopathic clinic need?
- Is homoeopathy able to be integrated with conventional approaches?
- How long do homoeopathic consultations need to be?

Several publications point out that homoeopathic treatment has lower costs than other treatments. This might be true. However, costs should not be considered before efficacy is accepted (see also under Practicability p. 28).

Prescribers' expertise
Education, training and examination of physicians and their staff is a problem common to all kinds of health providers. For homoeopathy questions arise such as:

- What training and qualifications does a homoeopath need?
- What level of qualification and experience is necessary for a homoeopath to run a practice or clinic with full responsibility?
- Is a medical qualification necessary for homoeopaths?
- How large is the inter-homoeopath variability in prescribing (e.g. for the same patient)? This can be investigated for homoeopaths of the same school and for members of different homoeopathic schools.

Qualification, examination, approval and supervision of homoeopaths are tasks within the homoeopathic community and should therefore be done by homoeopathic organizations and schools.

Improvement of homoeopathic strategies
Some of the questions which address improvement and optimization of homoeopathic procedures are:

- How long do homoeopathic consultations (case taking and follow-up) need to be?
- What are the psychological and psychosomatic effects of the elaborate history and case taking on patients?
- Which strategies lead to the most successful prescription?
- Which remedies give good clinical results?
- Which symptoms and prescribing data are most reliable and lead to the optimal remedy?
- What potencies are most effective and deliver the best therapeutic results?
- What dosage regimes give best clinical results?
- In which circumstances do unicist and/or multiple prescribing strategies yield the best results?

Usually the administration of the correct homoeopathic remedy is considered to be the reason for therapeutic success. Therefore, ascertaining this remedy for a particular patient, given his or her disease and his or her situation and lifestyle, is the homoeopath's most important task. A properly selected and prescribed homoeopathic remedy might have psychological and psychosomatic effects beyond those related to the pathology. This gives rise to questions such as:

- What are the psychological, psychosomatic, social benefits (and maybe risks) of homoeopathic treatment other than its clinical efficacy?

Especially for patients with trivial illnesses, psychosomatic disorders, and for patients with incurable diseases, homoeopathy might be a psychological and social help. But the authors think that these are the principal secondary questions which should be taken up after the question on efficacy of properly prescribed homoeopathic drugs has been answered (see also under Improvement of homoeopathic strategies p. 28).

Provings
Remedy provings are the most important source of drug pictures of the homoeopathic materia medica. They may be supplemented by toxicological data, and that from successful clinical experience, but they are essential for a full drug picture to be developed. A continuing supply of high quality provings is essential for the continuance of homoeopathy.

The drug picture is assessed by remedy proving by healthy volunteers. Questions concerning provings, the documentation of effects of substances producing symptoms in healthy people, are:

- Which symptoms occur after application of a certain remedy?
- Do the same symptoms occur with low and high potencies?
- How many subjects, which potencies and doses are needed in a proving?
- Are individual symptoms reproducible in cross-over designs and in different provings?
- How similar are symptoms of different individuals?

For study designs for provings see p. 29.

Applicability in day-to-day care
A further type of question deals with the problem how can homoeopathy be applied in day-to-day care. Questions arising in applicability in day-to-day care are:

- What side-effects or complications occur when prescribing homoeopathic remedies?
- Is homoeopathy in demand by patients and physicians?
- What is the level of such demand in different locations?
- Is homoeopathy meeting patients' and practitioners' expectations?
- Which instructions for case taking and remedy prescription should be given?
- How and to what extent should the patient be informed about the applied homoeopathic strategy?
- How compliant are patients?

See also p. 29.

Assessment of therapeutic success

For the assessment of therapeutic success one or more outcome variables have to be defined (see Outcome variables p. 32). In general in clinical research, primary and secondary outcome variables have to be distinguished. Whether an outcome variable is called a primary or a secondary outcome variable depends on its importance within the context of the research.

An important outcome variable evaluated by inference statistical methods will be called a primary outcome variable, while a less important variable not of primary interest is named a secondary outcome variable and is evaluated by explorative data analysis.

Overall, the superiority of a homoeopathic treatment could be expressed in all kinds of therapeutic success, in safety and in costs.

Efficacy

In clinical research efficacy is measured mostly by clinical variables. In studies on efficacy such outcome variables are used as primary outcome variables for the analysis of the data. Clinical outcome variables might be, for instance, blood pressure, grip strength, walking distance or relapse rate. If in a study the clinical endpoint is pain-relief, this can be measured by subjective evaluation of pain on a rating scale or a visual analogue scale. Alternatively it might be useful to measure therapeutic success by investigating the amount of allopathic medication consumed, e.g. analgesics. In this case the amount of allopathic medication is a surrogate endpoint for pain.

If in a study on classical homoeopathy the efficacy of a remedy at a high dilution can be demonstrated, this simultaneously leads to different interpretations. First there will be the interpretation of an effective particular drug and, second, study results will have established biological activity beyond Avogadro's number.

In classical homoeopathy the efficacy of a remedy depends on whether the individual clinical picture and drug picture are well-matched. This might be assessed by documentation of the homoeopath's degree of confidence in the prescription and subgroup analysis of the different degrees of confidence.

Benefit

Outcome variables measuring benefit are mostly secondary outcome variables, but they might also be the primary outcome variables of a study. The benefit of a therapy is completely defined by prolongation of life-span and quality of life. Nowadays, prolongation of life-span and/or improvement of quality of life is often thought to be more important for patients than to improve laboratory and other diagnostic measures. This is especially true for homoeopathy, which claims to improve the general health status of the patients. For treatments supposed to be equally effective, the comparison of benefits and risks will help to make a decision as to which treatment should be recommended.

Interviews and questionnaires are being used to measure quality of life. Several validated instruments are available (Guggenmoos-Holzmann *et al.*, 1995; Bullinger, 1991). Questionnaires have been developed for different diseases (e.g. cancer) addressing the peculiarities of these diseases.

Often in studies, on cancer for instance, the survival time is used to measure the therapeutic success. Alternatively, it might be more appropriate to document the time to recurrence of the tumour or to occurrence of complications. In general the failure time is the length of the time interval between e.g. diagnosis, surgery or the beginning of a particular treatment and the occurrence of a certain specified event. The observed times will be used for analysis and will be called uncensored observations. In the same way, a censored observation will be the similar time interval until the patient is lost to follow-up.

Patient satisfaction

Measurement of patient satisfaction might be used to compare treatments or to get an impression of the extent to which a particular treatment meets the patient's expectations. In this case, it will be necessary to measure the individual goal attainment on a pre-specified scale. The aim will be to standardize the individual goal attainment scale and make individual results comparable.

Patient satisfaction should be used as an additional outcome variable, i.e. a secondary outcome variable, if a clinical endpoint of interest is measurable. If on the other hand such an endpoint is not feasible or if therapies are equally effective it might be appropriate to evaluate therapies by an outcome variable based on patient satisfaction. Study designs focused on patient satisfaction are mentioned on p. 24 and p. 25.

Safety

Tolerability and safety have to be questioned for all kinds of therapies including homoeopathy. However, nobody has seriously claimed severe side-effects from homoeopathic remedies in medium or high potencies. None are documented in extensive literature searches. As long as an urgent treatment is not delayed or omitted, homoeopathy is regarded by most people as harmless and safe. However, if undesired events occur during or after homoeopathic treatment, especially under the conditions of a study, they have to be recorded, reported and discussed.

Tolerability and safety of a therapeutic approach is of great importance for every trial and study. During and after treatment it is mandatory to document adverse events. However, some adverse events might only be observed after long continued treatment. It will be important to distinguish between adverse drug reactions and adverse events occurring due to other reasons than application of the drug.

Cost-effectiveness

To evaluate cost-effectiveness and establish a cost-benefit ratio, efficiency has to be measured and the total cost has to be determined. Moreover it might be interesting to investigate savings in costs of conventional treatment by adding a homoeopathic therapy over the same time.

As already mentioned on p. 15, the question of the cost-effectiveness of homoeopathic remedies becomes important after efficacy is demonstrated. Homoeopathic remedies are assumed to be less expensive than allopathic remedies. If for example homoeopathic and conventional treatment are equally effective and the cost of the former is lower, homoeopathy might be chosen by the provider in preference to conventional therapy.

Types of studies

There are different types of studies and analysis strategies important for clinical research in homoeopathy (Gaus, 1990). Epidemiological studies such as cross-sectional, cohort or case-control studies might be appropriate at a first step. These three study types have in common that no intervention takes place and that patients are not randomized. A cross-sectional study is a survey to study the state of a population at a certain point of time. In a cohort study a large sample of individuals either exposed or not exposed to a certain risk factor or treatment is observed and the health status of the cohort members is recorded during subsequent years. A cohort study is a prospective study, but the beginning of the exposure or treatment may be in the past. A case-control study is a retrospective study: individuals with or without a certain disease are studied to analyse the frequency of explanatory variables for this disease.

Various types of clinical trials can be designed. They may differ with respect to randomization, open, single-masked or double-masked treatment, cross-over or parallel group design, single-centre or multi-centre trial, pilot or major study, sequential or fixed sample clinical trial. Some possible designs which are relevant for clinical research in homoeopathy will now be described.

Data collection

Data collection is the documentation of homoeopathic practice and its results. Details of consultations, diseases, treatments and/or costs will be collected as they are observed in day-to-day homoeopathic practice.

These data can be used to generate hypotheses and give valuable indicators for directions of new clinical research. They can help to develop specific research questions and to screen for appropriate outcome variables. Associations among diagnosis, remedy choice, symptoms and recorded outcome can be evaluated. Trends in prescribing may be analysed, practitioners' skills may be checked, treatment durations may be estimated. They are a source of information about 'cured symptoms' which can be used in daily practice. There might be symptoms never observed in provings which are found to correlate with successful use of a given remedy, thereby adding valuable information to the materia medica. Thus, data collection can be used to improve homoeopathic practice. However, it is not possible to make unbiased comparisons among different treatments.

Important disadvantages of data collections are many missing observations, undefined observations and measuring devices, irregular frequency and time points of observations, an undefined study population, and many confounders. On the other hand, data collections are cheap and many cases can be collected retrospectively as well as prospectively in a short time.

Observational studies

An observational study is a type of epidemiological study. Patients are not randomized but the study population is well defined. In this study factors such as the effect of different therapeutic regimes are observed according to an observation protocol. In an observation protocol, time points of observation, the variables to be observed or measured at each time point, and measuring devices and procedures are specified.

Particular attention has to be paid to the selection of study patients to avoid bias in estimation of effects. There are three possible types of bias: confounding, selection and observation bias. Confounding bias is caused by factors affecting the study outcome but which are not of primary interest. These confounding factors represent no main effects of the study. Selection bias is due to shortcomings in the definition of the study population and the sampling procedure. Observation bias is caused by differences in the precision with which outcomes are recorded, or a lack of objectivity in measuring and evaluating outcomes. Observational studies also do not permit an unbiased comparison to be made between different treatments but do allow an adjustment for confounding factors by application of multivariate statistical analysis.

Uncontrolled clinical studies

An uncontrolled clinical trial is a prospective study designed to assess the effects of a treatment on patients with a given medical condition. Patients will not be randomized to treatment groups since no control group is investigated. Uncontrolled clinical trials are observational studies and might for instance be used as a screening process, to investigate drug effects, to check prescribers' skills, to assess practicability of a treatment or for surveillance after application.

Pilot studies

Pilot studies are launched for planning purposes where information is needed before a major study is undertaken. They can be controlled (with a control group for comparison) or uncontrolled (without a control group) clinical trials of small sample size. Studies on the efficacy of homoeopathic treatment have to satisfy the specific demands of homoeopathy as well as requirements stated by the scientific community and universities. They are conducted for a number of reasons including:

(a) to estimate the acceptability of a study by patients, homoeopaths and scientists,
(b) to evaluate the practicality of the proposed method,
(c) to give a raw estimate of the treatment effect and its variability,
(d) to test the suitability of the assessment (outcome) criteria, and
(e) to test the feasibility of the proposed methodology.

Conducting and analysing a pilot study will help to decide whether a larger study is worthwhile. The pilot study will give more detailed information regarding how the main study should be designed, how the study population should be recruited, which outcome variable(s) should be chosen, its necessary minimum duration, and the number of patients needed to obtain a valid result.

Internal pilot studies

Unfortunately, the inclusion of the data of pilot studies in the final inference statistical analysis requires specific statistical methods. Such an inclusion is possible without problems of interpretation if the pilot study and main study are of the same design. In such a case the whole study (internal pilot study and main study) can be planned so as to allow interim analysis. This would enable the investigator to adapt the sample size after the interim analysis. The results of the first stage of the study (internal pilot study) will then be used to calculate the sample size needed in the second stage of the study (main study). The impact of such a procedure on the inferential test procedure has to be considered. Bauer and Köhne (1994) proposed a general method of analysis of clinical trials including interim analyses without compromising the overall significance level. A procedure for two- and three-stage designs is described. Data from the stages before and after the interim analysis have to be evaluated separately. The p-values for the different stages have to be combined in a particular way to control the overall significance level.

In spite of the considerable advantages of such adaptive methods, there exists the problem of estimation. If the same hypothesis is tested several times throughout the study, the influence of stopping rules and adaptations on the estimates is difficult to assess. Pooling the estimates of the study stages will give a biased estimate, since a second stage is only investigated if the result of the first stage is not satisfactory (not significant) and because the study is closed after the first stage and the estimate is final if the result of the first stage is fine (significant). Nevertheless, the application of adaptive methods – especially if, as in homoeopathy, information about effect size is often rare – can be reasonable (Bauer and Röhmel, 1995).

Cross-over and single case design

Cross-over design means that each patient will receive both (or more) treatments, one after the other with some time without either treatment in between. In contrast to cross-over, in a study with parallel groups each patient belongs either to treatment group A or B, one of which will be the verum, and one the placebo or a conventional treatment. The advantage of a cross-over design is that less patients are needed to compare the different study treatments, since each patient is his/her own control. However, there are also some drawbacks. Apart from the general problems of cross-over design (Brown, 1980; Jones and Lewis, 1995; Senn, 1995), such trials have the additional disadvantage (from the triallist's point of view) of lasting change in health resulting from an accurate homoeopathic prescription (see Control group on p. 34).

A trial with a single case design has only one individual patient and he or she is allocated a series of treatment periods (Guyatt *et al.*,1986). The sequence of treatments is randomized. Cross-over trials generally use a single cross-over from one treatment to the other but in a single case design multiple cross-overs are used. So periods of homoeopathic therapy and periods of conventional or placebo therapy are following in a random sequence. The treatment should be masked. Synonyms for single case design are 'intensive research design' and 'N of 1 design'.

A single case design shares many features with a common cross-over design. But the goal of an N of 1 trial is to investigate the efficacy of treatment for an individual patient, while a cross-over trial tries to establish a treatment effect for a population of patients. Although a meta-analysis for some N of 1 trials could be done, it is difficult to establish a treatment effect for a population. Treatments in the individual N of 1 trial are not standardized and the study population is difficult to specify. Special attention has to be paid for carry-over effects, i.e. the wash out phase between the treatment periods has to be long enough. Guyatt *et al.* (1990) propose N of

1 trials when developing new drugs. The aim is to get detailed knowledge of optimal dose, the most responsive patients and optimal outcome variables, which would be helpful when planning studies on the efficacy of a new drug.

Restrictions for conducting trials with single case design are similar to those of cross-over trials. The treatment should not be curative (otherwise a second period is unnecessary and unethical), the disease should be chronic or relatively stable, the treatment should have a rapid onset and should stop acting soon after it is discontinued, so the treatment effect does not carry over to the next treatment period, and treatment periods should be short (Guyatt *et al.*, 1988). Such studies might be possible in homoeopathy, and there is known interest in them. However, for treatment with a long-lasting success or with the hope to heal the patient completely – as in homoeopathy – neither single case design nor cross-over design is appropriate.

Randomized and strictly double-masked studies

Randomized studies with a control group and a certain degree of quality assurance are called controlled clinical trials (CCTs). CCTs, regardless of whether the therapies are masked or not, may be planned with cross-over design or parallel groups.

Randomized and strictly double-masked studies are highly recommended if possible. Considering the preceding specific methodological problems of homoeopathy, two proposals are given for conducting studies, one in classical homoeopathy and one in pathological prescribing.

In general, the efficacy of classical homoeopathic treatment with individual prescribing can be proven for a certain disease in a study designed in the following way. Patients are randomized to two treatment groups (A, homoeopathic treatment; B, placebo). Treatment under study is completely (double) masked. In the study the homoeopath will be allowed to prescribe any remedy in any potency at each consultation. Every patient gets an individualized treatment. If the patient belongs to treatment group A, he receives his individualized homoeopathic treatment. If the patient is randomized to group B, he gets a placebo looking like the prescribed homoeopathic remedy. To perform such a study a pharmacy could participate in the study and do the randomization and deliver all prescribed remedies – true medication as well as placebo – to the patients. It is no problem to have a stock of placebo-drops, placebo-globuli etc. in the study pharmacy. In the analysis the outcome variables of both groups will be compared to show efficacy of the homoeopathic treatment in general for the investigated diagnosis (Gaus, 1990, 1994). Such a study investigates the ability of homoeopaths to treat patients successfully. This design may be modified, to allow only a restricted choice of remedies.

For pathological prescribing the efficacy of a specific remedy can be proven if one specific syndrome described in detail can be used as an inclusion criterion of the study. For example patients with pollinosis or rheumatoid arthritis are randomized into one of two treatment groups in a double-masked CCT (Wiesenauer and Gaus, 1991; Wiesenauer and Lüdtke, 1995). Then, considering pathological prescribing the treatment for all study patients will be the same and proving efficacy means efficacy of the special study medication.

This type of study has been used to demonstrate that a 30C potency is not simply a placebo (Reilly *et al.,* 1986). In this study isopathy rather than homoeopathy was used. However, in the clinical application of a single remedy to a single disease entity, it is fundamental that the inclusion criteria include the clause that the patient's symptoms match the chosen remedy. In studies where this advice has not been followed (e.g. Shipley *et al.*, 1983) the results may be negative and meaningless, since the principles of homoeopathy have not been followed.

The first proposal for a study design takes into account the rules of classical homoeopathy such as individual remedy selection and the possibility of changing the medicine during the treatment. Additionally, it will be important to measure co-variables concerning the degree of suitability of the first prescription. The second proposal, however, fits pathological prescribing where the choice of both remedy and pathology is predetermined.

For more details on CCTs in homoeopathy see Controlled clinical trials in homoeopathy on p. 29.

Studies on equivalence

In some cases the objective of a study will be to demonstrate equivalence of homoeopathic and conventional therapy, e.g. in situations where using a placebo group would be unethical. The resulting hypothesis of the study would be that homoeopathy is equally effective (two-sided hypothesis) or at least as effective (one-sided hypothesis) as conventional therapy. These hypotheses cannot be answered by standard statistical methodology but by application of statistical tests on equivalence. For a study on equivalence a region of equivalence has to be specified before the study begins. Differences between treatments within the region of equivalence are defined as of minor importance, thus within this region the treatment effects are about the same and therefore equivalent.

Designing a clinical trial on equivalence will be done in the same way as designing other clinical studies. Treatment should be randomized and double-masked, no matter whether cross-over or parallel group design is used. However, sample size calculation and hypothesis testing have to be done in a specific way. Such trials might also pose considerable problems in interpretation because data can be biased towards equivalence even if the treatments are masked (Senn, 1993).

Studies with more than two parallel groups

In general clinical studies with two groups are conducted comparing homoeopathic medicine with placebo or a conventional therapy. However, if the aim of a study were to compare the efficacy of homoeopathic potencies compared with placebo and a conventional treatment, it would be appropriate to conduct a controlled clinical trial with more than two (parallel) groups.

In this situation special proposals for analysing the data, comparing study groups and proving efficacy are necessary. Evaluation could be done in a hierarchical way. That means that hypotheses are ordered to specify which hypothesis has to be evaluated or tested first, second, etc. The ordering of hypotheses will be done according to relevant medical and homoeopathic considerations. If a particular hypothesis can't be rejected, succeeding hypotheses may not be tested either. The sequence in which the hypotheses are tested has to be stated before the study begins (*a priori* ordered hypotheses) and has to be documented in the study protocol.

In any study with more than two (parallel) groups, the hypotheses to be tested have to be enumerated carefully. It is important to work out an appropriate strategy for comparing the groups. The statistical literature covers many more strategies for comparing more than two groups as mentioned here.

Option-to-continue and change-to-open-label design

An introductory approach to using patient satisfaction as a secondary outcome is to ask each patient at a time specified in the study protocol whether he wants to continue the (randomized, masked) therapy or not (option-to-continue design, Reilly *et al.*, 1994). If the patient decides to continue the study therapy this is considered as therapeutic success; if the patient decides not to continue the study therapy this is considered as therapeutic failure. A disadvantage of the option-to-continue design is its binary outcome variable, i.e. each patient delivers only one bit of information (bit = binary digit, the smallest amount of information in principle) and the power of the study is therefore rather small. The power of a statistical test is its ability to reject the null hypothesis if the alternative hypothesis is true. If for example two treatment groups have to be compared to demonstrate different therapeutic success, a statistical test can detect such a difference if it truly exists.

The change-to-open-label design (Högel, Walach and Gaus, 1994) overcomes this problem. Patients are randomized into treatment groups, whereby the treatment is masked. Patients are allowed to change to an unmasked treatment of their own choice if the study treatment is unsatisfactory. The main outcome variable is the time until a patient seeks a change in his/her treatment of his or her own choice. The data will be evaluated by survival analysis methods. The patient's impression of treatment success is most important and this determines the time until an open-label treatment is requested. The earlier a patient demands a change, the less satisfied he/she is with the study treatment. This design is especially suitable to investigate quality of life.

Optional cross-over design

The optional cross-over design (Ernst and Resch, 1995) could be applicable in situations where in a randomized CCT no 'hard' endpoint is available. The patients are randomized to treatments in phase 1. At the end of phase 1 the patients may change to the other treatment if they are dissatisfied, or continue with it if pleased. Further cross-over points may be considered later in the study. The outcome variable will be the proportion of patients treated with a certain treatment at the end of the study. If, for instance, homoeopathic treatment is equally effective as placebo, this will lead in the long run to 50 per cent of the patients receiving homoeopathic treatment and 50 per cent of the patients receiving placebo. If on the other hand homoeopathy is more effective than placebo, more patients will be in the homoeopathy group at the end of the study. Evaluation will be done applying the Chi-squared test of fit for 0.5:0.5.

Design with randomization option

The application of a design with a randomization option is appropriate if patients or their physicians are convinced of the efficacy of a particular therapy, e.g. homoeopathy. They want to decide whether they receive homoeopathic or allopathic therapy and they are not willing to be randomized. A way to consider patients' preference is to screen between patients preferring a certain therapy and those without a preference. Afterwards, patients with a preference will receive the requested therapy while others are randomized. This leads to four treatment groups:

- non-randomized patients with treatment A (e.g. homoeopathy)
- randomized patients with treatment A
- randomized patients with treatment B (e.g. conventional therapy)
- non-randomized patients with treatment B.

Patients can be allocated to a treatment group by their physician, for example. This design was proposed by Olschewski and Scheurlen (1985) to evaluate the external validity of a study and by Mau (1993) to allocate patients to two study centres applying different therapeutic therapies.

Studies investigating the influence of the study situation

To study whether the effects of homoeopathic treatment in daily practice differ from the effects measured in clinical trials and to study if the setting of a CCT with its patients' informed consent affects or even disturbs the homoeopathic case taking, remedy selection and therapeutic success, a randomized trial with five parallel groups is proposed. Differences between the study groups may occur due to the status of the patient, i.e. whether the patient knows that he is treated regularly homoeopathically (outside a clinical trial) or receives a homoeopathic remedy or placebo within a clinical trial. Further, treatment effects may depend on the status of the homoeopath. Different outcomes might be measured if the homoeopath definitely knows that the patient receives the homoeopathic remedy or if the homoeopath knows that the patient is randomized to the verum or the placebo group within a double-masked clinical trial.

Therefore, patients will be randomized to one of five parallel groups. These groups are defined as follows:

- group (A): both patient and therapist know that verum is applied (as in normal practice),
- group (B): the patient knows he is getting verum, but the therapist thinks it might be verum or placebo,
- group (C): the patient is told he might get either verum or placebo, but the therapist knows verum is supplied (single-masked therapy),
- group (D): the patient is given verum, but neither he nor the therapist know whether verum or placebo was delivered (double-masked therapy),

- group (E): the patient is given placebo, but neither he nor the therapist know whether verum or placebo was delivered (double-masked therapy).

Analysis of the results of these five groups will demonstrate whether and to which extent masking the treatment for the patient or the therapist will affect the outcome.

Application of designs and methods

Various types of study can be designed and many tools for analysis are available. Depending on the aim of research some designs are more or less appropriate. The following will summarize which methodology should be chosen to get answers to particular research questions.

Efficacy

Efficacy of a treatment (see p. 14) can only be demonstrated in a really convincing manner by a CCT (see pp. 29–45). These CCTs might be controlled by investigation of a placebo group or a group with conventional treatment, regardless of whether parallel groups or cross-over design (see p. 22) is chosen. A placebo control will be chosen if no standard therapy is established and if it is ethically acceptable. If not, an active control will be investigated.

In most situations a parallel group design is best (see p. 23). In situations where a conventional standard therapy is available and the use of placebo is not unethical, it might be appropriate to conduct a CCT with three parallel groups: one group receiving homoeopathic treatment, one group with conventional treatment and a placebo group. This will enable the investigator to demonstrate the efficacy of homoeopathy and its equivalence to the conventional therapy.

Randomization of patients to treatments and masking of treatments should be mandatory (see Randomization p. 34 and Guarantee of blindness p. 35). Randomization and masking will ensure structural, treatment and observational comparability. Structural comparability means that treatment groups do not have a different structure. All confounders, such as age, sex or severity of the disease, are identically distributed over treatment groups and differences between groups are only due to random effects. To obtain treatment comparability it is necessary to guarantee that all individuals are treated the same way except for the therapy itself. Observational comparability is ensured if certain rules are kept to examine patients, to evaluate therapeutic success, etc. For example, asking for adverse events has to be done as intensively in the placebo group as in the verum group. Structural, treatment and observational comparability are necessary to make study results easy to interpret. For instance, if treatment groups are not structurally comparable, differences in outcome could be caused by the treatment or by the different structure of the groups. Hence it is not known whether differences in outcome are due to different treatments or to the different demographic structures of the groups. Even if there is no difference in outcome a different therapeutic success (favouring e.g. group A) could have been compensated by a different structure of the treatment groups (e.g. favouring group B).

The problem of comparability of treatment groups may also complicate the interpretation of results of CCTs with a randomization option. Thus, the design with randomization option should only be applied if patients or their physicians are highly convinced of a particular therapy and it is not possible to randomize the patients. In this case the investigator should bear in mind that only the two randomized groups with patients without preference are comparable and that the other study results might be biased, difficult to interpret and equivocal.

Planning and designing CCTs often is complicated by the fact that detailed information is missing about e.g. eligible study patients, the size of the investigated effect, applicability of therapy and treatment duration. In this case, pilot studies are indicated, which should be designed in the same way as the main study, i.e. a CCT of smaller sample size.

Practicability

As already pointed out on p. 15, aspects of practicability might be assessed before, during or after efficacy has been demonstrated. Therefore, different study designs are appropriate. Data collections and observational studies may be used as well as CCTs.

If the spectrum of diseases treated by homoeopaths or the duration of homoeopathic consultations is of interest, data collection can be useful and an observational study can be conducted. Such a study might precede one on efficacy. On the other hand, costs of homoeopathic treatment and the possibility of its integration with conventional approaches should be investigated when or after efficacy is demonstrated. Thus, in CCTs some secondary outcome variables can be used to record the costs of treatment regimes, for example. But especially when efficacy has been demonstrated in a CCT, observational studies can be conducted to study long term effects (Walach *et al.*, 1994) to assess what facilities are needed and whether homoeopathy is able to be integrated with conventional medicine.

Improvement of homoeopathic strategies

There is a variety of questions on improvement of homoeopathy (see p. 16). Previously uninvestigated areas require a graded series of studies to explore them adequately. The first approaches might be observation and data collection studies, with the aim of generating more precise questions suitable for subsequent CCTs.

Provings

Provings are needed to develop new remedies and to clarify and improve knowledge of existing ones (see p. 17). Here the same arguments as for demonstrating efficacy apply (see p. 27). Both cross-over and parallel group design are appropriate (Walach, 1993; Koenig *et al.*, 1987). The place of placebo in provings remains undecided, and itself merits further research. Ethical questions have arisen in recent years but no proving is continued to the point when real damage to a proband is likely. There should therefore be no ethical restraint on well-designed proving studies.

The use of single case design can be discussed. However, a single N of 1 trial will not be sufficient to assess the drug picture. More N of 1 trials will be necessary which can be evaluated together to generate hypotheses. But this ends up in a study design similar to a CCT with cross-over design. In a single case design in general there are many more periods and cross-overs. Since in provings it will be more interesting to estimate inter-person variability than intra-person variability, it will be more efficient to conduct a placebo controlled cross-over trial with many patients than a small number of N of 1 trials with many periods of cross-over.

Applicability in day-to-day care

Applicability of a therapy in day-to-day care (see p. 17) covers aspects which can be looked at by data collection or observational studies. Data collection may have the advantage of a long follow-up time already available if the data base has been established a long time ago. This is important if the tolerability and safety of therapies are studied. Observational studies can record patients' treatment and the healing process prospectively with a standardized observation scheme and data can be collected over a long follow-up time. Accurate definition of a study population can then lead to more valid results.

Controlled clinical trials (CCTs) in homoeopathy

Necessity of a control group

There are different reasons for treatment success under placebo:

- Improvement or spontaneous healing may occur due to its catalytic effect on the self-healing power of the body.
- Beside drugs, therapy consists of many components such as nursing, rest, counselling, etc. These components also contribute to therapeutic success.
- Elimination of environmental hazards, stress and reduction of daily problems will also help. Hahnemann recognized these when he spoke of 'obstacles to cure', which are certainly relevant and should be looked for where therapy fails, either in daily clinical practice or in the course of a clinical trial.
- The onset of therapy is at or after the climax of the disease, which in the course of its natural history was going to get better anyway.
- Finally, there might be a placebo effect in its narrow meaning, i.e. the belief and confidence of the patient that the physician and his therapy can support the healing process.

Therefore, it is necessary to have a control group in each study (Gaus, 1993). Consequently, case reports and studies without a control group (uncontrolled studies) can only be used to generate hypotheses.

To demonstrate the efficacy of homoeopathic medication, some patients will receive a homoeopathic remedy and others get placebo. A comparison of homoeopathic treatment success and treatment success under placebo can be performed. Alternatively, patients in the control group might receive conventional therapy when the disease under investigation has to be treated and placebo is inappropriate on ethical grounds (see also p. 34). In such a study equivalence of therapies will be the alternative hypothesis which is to be verified.

To ensure internal validity, i.e. that observed differences in treatment success between the two treatment groups truly result from the different therapies, the groups have to be comparable in their structure (composition), treatment (except the topic under investigation) and in the observations made on them. The tools to achieve structural comparability are randomization and stratification. In a randomized trial patients are allocated randomly to the treatment groups, whereby for each patient the chance of receiving treatment A (e.g. homoeopathic remedies) or treatment B (e.g. placebo) is equal. Comparability in treatment and observation can be achieved by investigating a control group, using placebo, and by masking the therapies for the patient and the physician. In a double-masked study, neither patient nor physician know to which study group the patient belongs. Consequently, all observations including assessment of treatment success cannot be biased by personal attitudes and beliefs. Nevertheless, the double-blind method has been criticized as introducing bias as a result of the blinding procedure itself (Kiene, 1996). For counter-arguments to this, see Studies investigating the influence of the study situation p. 26.

Outline of CCTs

Many aspects have to be considered when planning, conducting and evaluating a CCT. Some basic questions should be thoroughly addressed when planning a clinical trial (Reilly and Taylor, 1993), especially in homoeopathy, and when writing the study protocol. Essentials for all stages are listed below.

- A simple question and a clear aim of the study are necessary to get a clear answer.
- A control group must be included, if efficacy is to be proven.
- Therapists' skills have to be demonstrated.
- Before recruiting a patient for the study the inclusion and exclusion criteria have to be checked, the patient's informed consent has to be obtained, the admission of the patient to the study has to be documented and then, and not before, the patient is randomized.
- In a double-masked study, the active remedy and placebo must be indistinguishable for patients and physicians.
- The quality of all trial medicaments must be assured.
- Necessary investigations and procedures to be carried out at each visit must be laid out beforehand.

- Examinations should take place at scheduled time intervals. An appropriate programme of interviews, questions, procedures and investigations should be defined for each visit.
- Well-defined, accepted and previously validated outcome variables are necessary. Primary and secondary outcome variables have to be distinguished as well as hypothesis generation and hypothesis testing. A hypothesis, which needs to be tested by a CCT, must be generated before the CCT begins and must be stated very clearly in the protocol.
- Case report forms have to be specially developed for each study. They should reflect the investigations of each visit.
- Monitoring and data checking has to be performed by an independent person from outside the hospital or clinic.
- A statement confirming that the regulations of European Good Clinical Practice (GCP) guidelines are being followed.
- The evaluation of the trial and the biometrical report must contain the following:
- – a deposit of the source data gained by the study, preferably computerized,
  – a description of irregularities in performing the study, deviations from the study protocol, completeness and quality of data,
  – a description of the study patients, and as a consequence, a description of the population to which the study results apply,
  – an analysis of drop-outs and a description and assessment of comparability of groups,
  – an evaluation of the primary outcome variable(s), including descriptive statistics, estimations and testing of the hypotheses under investigation,
  – an evaluation of secondary outcome variables, explorative data analysis, generation of new hypotheses,
  – analysis of undesired events and safety,
  – assessment of the validity of study results.

Eligibility criteria

A clinical trial investigates a certain disease or complaints. Obviously, the lower the confidence in the diagnosis and the milder the disease and its complaints, the easier therapeutic success is achieved. Hence, in all therapeutic trials the certainty of diagnosis and severity of disease and complaints have to be defined, observed and recorded. Certainty of diagnosis and severity of disease and complaints are relevant for the interpretation of the results of the study.

The population investigated by a clinical study is defined by inclusion and exclusion criteria. Often used inclusion criteria are specific diagnoses, certain symptoms, a pathological result in a specified diagnostic procedure, the aetiology of the disease, a defined range of severity of the disease and its symptoms, etc. Often used exclusion criteria are age under 18 (for legal reasons), pregnancy (to save the unborn), severe concurrent disease or medication (to exclude a possible interaction of diseases or therapies), the expectation of non-compliance of the patient, etc. All recruited patients must fulfil all inclusion, and have no exclusion criteria.

In planning a study the relative width of inclusion and exclusion criteria needs to be addressed. Larger sample sizes are easier to obtain with wide criteria, but wide criteria introduce more heterogeneity among the patients. The decision will also depend on whether the results of the study should be valid for many persons (wide inclusion and exclusion criteria) or if the investigated therapy acts upon a specific group of patients (narrow criteria).

From the legal point of view patients eligible for a clinical trial have to be informed on their disease, the study and its therapies (including randomization, masking of treatments, placebo, etc. if used), alternative therapies outside the study, chances and risks of all possible therapies and the patients' rights (participation in the study is voluntary and may be cancelled at any time without giving a reason). Then the informed patient may give consent to participate in the study. Obviously, given informed consent by the patient is an inclusion criterion.

Outcome variables

A time-frame should be stated in which a therapeutic improvement is expected. In homoeopathy a long term follow-up period will often be necessary, since it claims improvement in the long run. Besides, considerations about the feasibility of the study will determine the treatment duration. With regard to measuring efficacy and complete healing the treatment duration is likely to be longer, but on grounds of feasibility a short treatment duration will often be chosen. These reflections will lead to determination of the treatment duration and a clear definition of the time the outcome variable is measured. It is vital that feasibility considerations should not be given precedence over the legitimate requirements of the study and lead to bad studies with uncertain results.

In each clinical study therapeutic success has to be defined and outcome variables measuring it must be established. For primary and secondary outcome variables see Assessment of therapeutic success p. 17. The following proposals may help for an objective and valid assessment of the therapeutic success achieved.

The assessment of therapeutic success should be done by a homoeopath as well as by a conventional physician to get a valid measurement of the outcome. Ideally they should agree on the achieved therapeutic success of each patient. As far as possible widely accepted outcome variables and validated measuring instruments should be used. In certain situations and for some outcome variables (e.g. pain, well-being, satisfaction) the patient's opinion might be more important than the doctor's opinion. Therefore, the patient's opinion should be considered when assessing therapeutic success.

Alternatively, the assessment of therapeutic success of each patient may be done by a competent and outstanding person not directly involved in the study therapy. To get a valid measurement of the outcome variable(s) it will be necessary to mask the treatment and to investigate a placebo group, a group receiving homoeopathic therapy and possibly a group receiving conventional therapy. Masking of the study therapies and the investigation of an additional parallel group with conventional therapy will avoid underestimation of the matter under investigation, which might be likely if only two groups (placebo and homoeopathic treatment) are considered. This will help to make the outcome measure acceptable for homoeopathy as well as for conventional medicine.

Diaries should be filled out by the patient or by the parents of the patient, if children are investigated. Outcome variables from these diaries often build the basis to prove efficacy.

Another possible way of demonstrating efficacy of homoeopathic treatment is the reduction of allopathic medication, e.g. analgesics, drugs for lowering blood pressure, or corticosteroids.

Measuring quality of life is also an appropriate outcome variable. Patients' well-being or quality of life should be investigated in almost all studies. It allows comparisons between therapies which are equally effective but have different adverse drug reactions. This is important because homoeopathic therapy often has fewer adverse drug reactions than conventional therapy. The questionnaire for measuring quality of life should be well and widely accepted or validated before its application (Bullinger, 1991; Guggenmoos-Holzmann, 1995).

Outcome measures must relate to the purposes of the treatment, so in classical homoeopathy they must measure well-being and general health as well as parameters related to pathology. For this purpose a quality of life measure will be appropriate.

Outcome variables measuring patient satisfaction might be constructed by determination of individual treatment goals. In this case the outcome variable describes the individual goal attainment measured on a pre-specified scale.

Sometimes, the clinical endpoint is too difficult or too expensive to measure, so suitable intermediate or surrogate outcome variables have to be chosen to replace it. In a study about, for instance, the prevention of the atherosclerosis by application of blood lipid-lowering drugs the clinical endpoint 'artherosclerosis' may be replaced by the intermediate endpoint 'decrease of blood cholesterol level'. An appropriate surrogate outcome variable should satisfy three basic requirements (Boissel *et al.*, 1992):

- it should occur more often than the corresponding clinical endpoint,
- the relationship between surrogate and clinical endpoint should be well established,
- an estimate of the expected clinical benefit should be derivable from the estimate of the reduction of the surrogate outcome variable.

Unfortunately there is often insufficient information available to validate the surrogate endpoint, so the above criteria cannot always be met.

Attention has to be paid to confounders, that is, factors which might alter or even disturb (amplify or reduce) the effects of treatment. For instance, co-interventions must be avoided or allowed for, and randomization must be stratified for important covariates to ensure structural equality and comparability of treatment groups. Otherwise, study results are difficult to interpret.

Control group
The necessity of a control group has already been discussed on p. 29. The inclusion of placebo control group should always be considered to enable adjustment for psychological and other factors in homoeopathic treatment. In this respect, the design will be similar to studies in conventional medicine. Additionally or as an alternative, if a placebo group is impossible on ethical grounds, the control group may be a cohort of patients treated with conventional therapy alone.

The most appropriate design to demonstrate efficacy is a controlled clinical trial with parallel groups. Standard cross-over trials are usually inappropriate for clinical studies in homoeopathy, because homoeopathic treatment claims protracted effects and lasting changes in health (Lange-deKlerk *et al.*, 1995), which affects the group of patients who start by receiving verum and progress to receiving the control treatment: the duration of the normally included wash-out phase would be impossible to calculate.

Recruitment
Not all patients suffering from the disease under investigation may be suitable for homoeopathic therapy. After adequate consultation the homoeopath might conclude that it is not possible to select an effective homoeopathic remedy for a particular patient with any confidence. This ought to be an legitimate exclusion criterion. Where patients are admitted to a trial, the homoeopath will still have a range of degrees of confidence in the prescription. In some studies, it might be appropriate to take account of this by analysing the results for subgroups with high prescription confidence and for subgroups with low prescription confidence.

Patients may be recruited from homoeopaths' practices, specialist clinics or through public advertisement. However, when patients are recruited through public media there is the risk that many patients with long histories of chronic diseases will be harder to treat successfully while highly motivated patients will be easier to treat. From the methodological point of view there are no objections to recruitment through public media, because all groups (homoeopathic, conventional and placebo treatment) are affected the same way. Further, if patients are recruited this way larger sample sizes are possible and a significant result of the study would be highly convincing.

Randomization
Randomization is compulsory to ensure structural comparability of treatment groups. It should be done by an independent person outside the hospital or clinic, not directly involved in the clinical part of the study. The randomization plan should be deposited with an independent body to ensure that therapies are masked for patient and physician. Moreover, it is necessary that each randomization is documented at time of randomization.

If confounders are known affecting the therapeutic success, it is important to use stratified randomization. The randomization will be stratified by those confounders known or expected to be the most important. The aim is to eliminate as many sources of bias as possible. Application of this technique should lead to treatment groups of the same structure with respect to the distribution of the confounders. For example, patients might be stratified according to the severity of their disease or any other variable which reduces heterogeneity of the population and defines homogenous subgroups. In multi-centre trials randomization should be done by a central secretariat and if each physician represents one study centre, randomization should be stratified by the physicians to minimize the effect of the physician, his/her practice or centre and to make treatment groups comparable. In some cases telefax is an excellent medium for randomization. Computer-based randomization is another possibility.

Guarantee of blindness

Working with masked study therapies is essential in any study to ensure treatment comparability and observational comparability. The demonstration of genuine blindness should therefore be an important aspect of a CCT. This is especially true in homoeopathy because any positive study result will be seriously questioned by conventional physicians disposed to doubt it, and any negative result by homoeopaths looking for an explanation of failure. Usually the randomization plan is instigated and administered by the study's biometrician. Once prepared, it should be deposited with a reputable independent person (trustee) so that there is no possibility of falsifying the results. When the study is done, all source data should be deposited with the code holder or even in a public domain file before de-masking is done for evaluation of the data. This would be an extremely strict and safe procedure to ensure that results of the study are true.

Rules have to be laid down for de-masking the therapy of an individual patient during study, if this should become necessary, e.g. in case of emergency. Normally de-masking of therapy is not allowed until the end of the entire study, when the treatment code is de-masked for evaluation and interpretation.

De-masking for evaluation can be done in two steps. In the first step it is released which patients are in the same group, say group X and group Y, but it is still unknown whether patients belonging to group X or group Y got true medication or placebo. Then the complete statistical evaluation is done and deposited or even published. Finally, as the second step of de-masking, it will be specified whether patients of group X or group Y received verum or placebo.

Prescribers' expertise and skills

This section will begin by examining the different level of skill that may be required in studies, then consider how they may be assured: through education, and through scientific verification.

Different forms of homoeopathic intervention require different levels of prescribers' skills. This applies to the three stages of (a) remedy selection, (b) administration regime chosen (i.e. the number and frequency of repetitions chosen), and (c) follow-up monitoring.

The different models of remedy selection may be considered as a spectrum from:

- **Complex homoeopathy** – This employs mixtures of drugs used for specific clinical indications, e.g. migraine, hay fever. This requires little or no homoeopathic diagnostic skill, but the clinician will need instructions in the issues of how the patient should take the remedy, and simple aspects of case management, e.g. how to deal with an apparent aggravation of symptoms. The clinician will require the conventional skills determined by the clinical problem under test, and that is true of the other models which follow.
- **Single remedy indications** – e.g. a pollen potency in hay fever, colocynthis in infant colic. A similar requirement plus a simple understanding of modalities and case follow-up (see algorithms below).
- **Algorithm prescribing** – Repertorization can use modern techniques like algorithms and computer programs. Matching of remedy pictures and patients' symptoms can be done by computer. Indeed, there are computer applications for prescribing individual homoeopathic remedies. None of these computer systems are widely accepted by leading homoeopaths, and the method itself would need scientific evaluation before being accepted or rejected. This is clearly a research question which may follow later, and not one of immediate concern. As more commonly understood, algorithm prescribing allows the prescriber a limited list of homoeopathic drugs from which the prescription must come. The prescriber must have the skill to do this, and the degree of skill must relate to the size of the limited list. Those patients whose symptoms do not suggest one of these remedies must be excluded from the trial. This has the two disadvantages of disappointing patients who have volunteered, adding to recruitment problems, and tempting the prescriber to make inaccurate prescriptions because he/she wants to obtain enough patients for the trial. These temptations and risks have been reported (verbally) by clinicians involved in such trials, which for these reasons are not recommended. Additionally prescribers' skills are also necessary because the homoeopath, not the algorithm, has to do the case taking including the anamnestic talk, the observation and characterization of patients' symptoms, an assessment of findings and, as a consequence, the steering of the talk with the patient towards his problems relevant for diagnosis and prescribing. All these processes are highly dependent on the skills of the homoeopath. Therefore, algorithms and computer programs may replace a printed book for repertorization, but not prescribers' skills.

For algorithm prescribing four different stages can be defined:

- **Simple algorithms:** Unless the selection criteria are really just normal medical ones, the use of these algorithms will normally require the prescriber to have an introductory level training in homoeopathy to understand for example the principal of individualized care and methods of eliciting and judging these modalities.
- **Moderately complicated algorithms with prescriber guidelines:** These require moderate degrees of homoeopathic training, for example Primary Health Care Certificate level (see education models below).

- **Complex algorithms:** These require full ability to diagnose the homoeopathic drug picture. Even if a study has a restricted remedy list, this will require full homoeopathic skill, equivalent to specialist status (see below). A good scientific reason for restricting the normal specialist's prescribing repertoire should be given.
- **Fully individual homoeopathy:** This requires full specialist training and skill in the given school of homoeopathy being employed.

In homoeopathy therapeutic success has two pre-requisites: prescribers' skills and action of prescribed remedies. A study on success of homoeopathic treatment investigates a complex of prescribers' skills and drug action. Demonstration of prescribers' skills is therefore necessary for all homoeopaths participating in the study before the study begins.

There are different sorts of evidence which might be offered within a study protocol in support of the claim that both 'active ingredients', i.e. the prescribers' skills and remedy action, are sound prior to the study. To help judge their worth, prescribers' skills could perhaps be evaluated in a hierarchy of reliability.

- Historic use of and/or confidence in the prescriber(s) is the least reliable. From the scientific point of view this should be taken as unproven.
- Certified skills such as completion of foundation training or specialist training (see below) are an important starting point, but not an ending point, of the process of verfication of prescribers' skill.
- Field-tested skills using techniques such as mock histories, video presentation and evaluation by a panel of experts are of value but less so (and potentially more complex) than the next stages.
- Evidence of general homoeopathic competence, demonstrated in e.g. a supervised data collection programme.
- Prescribers' skills can also be demonstrated in a pilot study. In the pilot study a smaller sample of patients would be treated with the method in the study protocol but without a placebo control. This has a further advantage of testing the outcome methods, their timing, their reliability and their validity.

Researchers and protocol reviewers should thus consider if there is a need for an initial 'feasibility enquiry' as it may be the best way to test the prescribers' skills and the proposed treatment model, before continuing on to the controlled trial. False negative results from inadequate treatment models and prescribers' skills will thus be avoided.

There is no unified Europe-wide certification at this time, and although it is recommended that protocols are developed and reviewed by teams including someone who can give a competent opinion on the qualifications of the homoeopathic prescribers, it must be recognized that it can be difficult to judge.

That said, consensus has been reached on the requirement for programmes of homoeopathic training standards for medical doctors, and there are a number of published guidelines.

- The European Committee for Homoeopathy gives in its report *Homoeopathy in Europe 1994* the basic training required of a specialist homoeopath.
- In the UK the Faculty of Homoeopathy membership exam (MFHom) is the most established of the specialist post-graduate examinations with many decades of development and experience. It was the template for some parts of the report *Homoeopathy in Europe 1994*. The Faculty of Homoeopathy has now published a clinical standards document outlining the addition requirements beyond the post-graduate examination to become a specialist (The Faculty of Homoeopathy, 1995).
- Many studies could employ prescribers with skills less than those of full specialists. Here the UK Faculty of Homoeopathy's new Primary Health Care Certificate in Basic Homoeopathy (PHCC) which is obtained after one year of study and an examination, offers a model for basic level skill (Reilly, 1994, 1995).

Repeated prescriptions

One of the difficulties of homoeopathic practice is to find the remedy that most closely matches the individual and his/her clinical picture. This is especially true at the first consultation, when the doctor knows the patient least well. It is therefore sometimes necessary to choose another remedy at a later consultation.

Alternative designs could be suggested which allow for de-masking. Patients could be randomized a second or third time after the code was broken. There might be two approaches: one involving further randomization of patients at a pre-specified time point no matter whether treatment was successful or not, another only allowing de-masking and re-randomization of unsuccessful patients.

These designs have their own serious problems. In the first design analysis might be complicated by having more groups than treatments, e.g. treatment A, then treatment B; treatment A, then again treatment A; treatment B, then treatment A; treatment B, then again treatment B. If analysed this way the statistical analysis is bound to be less powerful. Assessment of success is difficult if patients receive placebo and verum in randomized order, especially when the prolonged effect of homoeopathic medicines is taken into account.

The second design may lead to unequal sample sizes in the treatment groups, another cause of loss of power. The estimates for main effects will be biased because only unsuccessful treatment is de-masked and only these patients are randomized a further time. It is possible to overestimate the difference between verum and placebo because responders are selected to the verum group.

These considerations lead to the recommendation that, where efficacy in a clinical situation is the question to be answered, the standard design of a placebo-controlled double-masked clinical trial is the trial of choice, since despite its drawbacks, it is more reliable and enjoys better credibility within the scientific community. If a patient has no success in a placebo-controlled double-masked clinical trial and the homoeopath wonders whether he/she has prescribed the right remedy, he/she should assume that each patient belongs to the verum group. If the patient is really in the verum group this strategy is correct, if not, this strategy does no harm. This strategy minimizes bias in this respect. Additionally, the number of prescriptions could be analysed as a secondary outcome variable. In the placebo group more changes would be expected.

Drop-outs, withdrawals

It is clearly desirable to achieve as low a drop-out rate as possible because drop-outs reduce not only the sample size and therefore the power of the study, but can introduce bias and disturb the comparability of groups. However, in any trial some patients will drop out. It will be important for data analysis to document all their reasons for doing so, which might be therapy related or not.

In homoeopathy, as has been discussed, there may be an initial aggravation at the beginning of the treatment, which causes some patients to drop out despite receiving prior warning, although skilled explanation and coaching should reduce this number.

Conversely it is known from homoeopathic trials that some patients fail to follow-up because they are so much better that they do not want to waste time seeing their doctor. To assume a poor result because the patient gave no reason for his non-return may actually be inaccurate. Therefore, the effort to establish the reason for withdrawal is important.

Analysis of data should be based on the 'intention-to-treat' principle. According to this principle all patients have to be included in the analysis regardless whether they withdrew, were lost to follow-up, were treated according or not according to protocol. If no outcome data are available for drop-outs and the reason for withdrawal of the treatment is not clarified, a poor therapeutic success should be assumed for intention-to-treat evaluation.

Additionally, a second analysis may be performed following the principle 'according-to-protocol', i.e. only patients treated and observed according to protocol are included in the evaluation. Study results will only be valid if the intention-to-treat analysis and the according-to-protocol analysis yield internally consistent results. Otherwise, all study results have to be interpreted very carefully and restrictively.

Sample size determination

In statistics there are well-known formulae and procedures to estimate the sample size of a study (Lachin, 1981; Pocock, 1983). The sample size (this is the number of evaluable patients per group) mainly depends on:

- **The type of outcome variable.** A quantitative outcome variable delivers most information from each patient, while a binary outcome variable delivers least information. Hence, for a study with a binary outcome variable many more patients are required than for a study with a quantitative outcome variable.
- **The design of the study.** A cross-over design – if really justified – requires a lower sample size than a parallel group design.

- **The number of statistical tests for confirmatory hypothesis testing.** If only one test is done, the level of significance and therefore the power is focused on this test. The more tests are done, the more the level of significance and the power is divided and each test has only a small chance to become significant. Therefore, the more tests for confirmatory hypothesis testing are scheduled, the more patients are needed.
- **The number of treatment groups.** Having more than two groups has the disadvantage of increasing the total number of patients needed for the study, because the power of a study is based on the number of patients per group.
- **The assumed minimal differences between groups.** Where only minor differences between groups are detected, large samples are necessary. When only large differences are to be detected small samples suffice.
- **The hypotheses to be tested.** One-sided hypotheses need fewer patients to become significant than two-sided hypotheses. However, there should be a very clear indication beforehand that one-sided testing is justified.
- **The level of significance.** A 1 per cent level of significance needs more patients than a 5 per cent level.
- **The power of the study.** Power is the probability of getting a significant result, provided a difference between the groups exists in reality. The larger the power should be the more patients are needed.

If a placebo group is investigated, attention has to be paid to the therapeutic success with placebo (see under Necessity of a control group on p. 29) to avoid over-optimistic assumption of the difference between the treatment groups for the sample size calculation.

Quality control of remedies and placebos

The quality of all trial medicaments must be assured. The homoeopathic remedies used in a CCT have to be produced according to Good Manufacturing Practice for Pharmaceutical Products (1992). The quality of raw materials, the name of their manufacturer, the details of their preparation, the name of their supplier and the potencies used must all be stated, certified correct and inspected by outside authorities.

Study protocol

The following recommendations should be used as a framework for planning new studies and the evaluation of already published studies in homoeopathy.

- All clinical studies in homoeopathy should be conducted according to GCP (Good Clinical Practice, 1991), GHCP (Good Homoeopathic Clinical Practice; European Committee for Homoeopathy, 1995) and the Declaration of Helsinki (Declaration of Helsinki, last revision, Hong Kong 1989).
- A clear and detailed study protocol should be worked out beforehand. The sponsor, the clinically responsible investigator and the biometrician must agree on, sign and date the protocol. Any alteration or supplement has to be written down as a formal amendment.

- The approval of an independent protocol review committee should be obtained. This committee should contain experts in conventional scientific medicine as well as homoeopaths so as to ensure that the results of the study may be accepted by the scientific community as a whole.
- Ethical approval must be obtained from the appropriate local ethical committee(s), according to GCP and the Declaration of Helsinki.
- Protocols of major studies should be deposited at a lawyer's office, or with a suitable responsible independent person, or be published beforehand. Where such exists, they should be registered with a central research registry before the study begins.
- The intention to publish the study results should be affirmed regardless of the results.

The study protocol is a detailed description of the planned study (Hulley and Cummings, 1988; Pocock, 1983) and should contain information at least about the following items.

- **General information.** The study protocol should contain the title of the project, the names of the clinically responsible investigators, all other investigators, the biometrician, monitors, sponsors and the place(s) where the trial will take place.
- **State of research and aim of study**. A review of previous relevant research and results of former studies must be described. Scientific and ethical arguments in support of conducting the new study must be given. The aim of the study must be presented in detail. The study protocol should include a clear and simple question to be answered by the study, formulated as null- and alternative hypothesis.
- **Design of the study.** The type of the study and its design must be specified (controlled study, pilot study, etc.) in detail. The randomization method and how randomization is arranged has to be described. The masking technique and how masking of treatments is guaranteed has to be laid down.
- **Definition of study population.** Reasons for the definition of the study population should be given. Inclusion and exclusion criteria have to be formulated adequately (e.g. age, sex, diagnostic admission criteria, certainty of diagnosis, patients' informed consent) and should be accepted by all concerned. Inclusion and exclusion criteria should be precise and leave no doubt about which patients may participate in the study and which may not. Recruitment methods must be specified.
- **Definition of patient visits, observation programme, and treatment.** The study protocol should go into detail about the length of, and interval between, doctor–patient consultations, the procedure to be followed at each consultation, including history-taking, examination of any diary which has been kept by participants, physical examinations and investigations which are necessary to conform the requirements of standard assessment proper to the clinical topic under investigation. These should be the standard, recognized, validated instruments agreed by conventional experts in the field. For each consultation the variables to be measured,

observed and documented have to be established. If necessary the measuring devices and conditions of measuring and observation should be described. The case report form for each visit reflects the variables to be observed and documented. The placebo must be specified and the chosen homoeopathic medicine, its potency and dose at each consultation and the dosage instructions for it, must be recorded, together with any concomitant treatment recommended.

- **Definition of study endpoints.** Primary and secondary outcome variables must be specified. They should be reliable, valid, and if possible quantitative. The time of measuring and how outcome variables are measured must also be defined.
- **Drop-outs.** Differentiation should be made between subjects who withdraw from the study and those who are lost to follow-up. A clear description of how to deal with them when analysing the study must be given.
- **Sample size and power.** The number of patients planned to be included must be stated. Reasons for the choice of the sample size must be given concerning power and clinical justification.
- **Biometric analysis.** The study protocol should contain the strategy for biometric evaluation and a list of the proper statistical methods to be employed.

Copies of explanatory letters to patients and case report forms should be available in an appendix to the protocol.

Performance and quality assurance

Multi-centre trials

In homoeopathy, recruiting many patients within a short time is often only possible if several physicians and/or homoeopaths agree to participate. Under these circumstances each physician or homoeopath represents a study centre. Homoeopathic multi-centre studies are highly desirable, although they have additional difficulties, as is well-known in conventional medicine (Gaus, 1993; Senn, 1995).

Therefore an important aspect to consider is variability between centres, especially inter-homoeopath variability. The study must assure a high quality of the homoeopathic prescriptions. To reduce inter-homoeopath variability the prescription might be supervised by a group of homoeopaths, or a conference of homoeopaths involved in the study might be arranged, where consensus is likely to be achieved. The homoeopaths' credentials, experiences and skills should be checked beforehand (see p. 35). Only well trained and experienced homoeopaths should participate (a minimum of five years' clinical homoeopathic experience has been suggested, some of which is in the field of investigation). The prescribing policies should be stated and agreed upon. By this means similar prescribing procedures and results may be achieved in all centres in spite of having different physicians involved.

Inter-homoeopath variability could be estimated in a pilot study. An anamnesis, including a description of the patient, the symptoms and diagnosis could be sent to several homoeopaths. Each homoeopath returns a prescription, so all prescribed remedies can be compared. However, this comparison will be complicated because even different remedies could be effective, and by the fact that reading someone else's patient history is a far cry from taking it one's self.

GCP regulations

The aim of GCP is to ensure that the rights and integrity of the trial subjects are thoroughly protected, to establish the credibility of data and study results, and to improve the ethical, scientific and technical quality of trials (CPMP Working Party, 1991). The GCP regulations give a lot of guidance on how to plan, perform and evaluate clinical studies. Quality is assured if GCP regulations are followed from planning a study to writing the final report.

Before and during a study the protection of the trial subjects has to be realized. Quality assurance covers, among other topics, the following issues:

- **Study protocol.** (See Study protocol p. 37.)
- **Case report forms.** A set of case report forms must be developed to document information on the patients in concordance with the study protocol. They are established to facilitate observation of the subjects. Aspects of security (e.g. adverse events) must be able to be documented.
- **Informed consent.** Patients' informed consent has to be obtained prior to inclusion in the trial but only after comprehensive oral or written information about the study including an explanation of its objectives, its purpose, the treatment (which might be active drug treatment or placebo), possible outcomes, potential benefits and risks, inconveniences, the patients' rights (e.g. the right to withdraw from the trial) and responsibilities according to the Declaration of Helsinki.

The investigator is an appropriately qualified person legally allowed to practice homoeopathy, is trained and experienced in research, particularly in the clinical area of the proposed trial, is familiar with the background to and the requirements of the study, and is known to have high standards of ethical and professional integrity.

After preparation of a draft version of the study protocol by the investigators and the biometrician the clinically responsible investigator has to review the protocol. The case report form and the documents for giving informed consent are prepared thereafter in accordance with the study protocol. Afterwards legal regulations for conducting the study are checked, and ethical committee approval is obtained.

Quality assurance during the study considers the whole range of protocol items from the correctness of patients' informed consent, to questions about medical care, controlling adherence to the study protocol, protection of privacy of the personal data, and ethical considerations. Amendments of the study protocol have to be proved necessary. Interim analysis might be planned according to ethical and statistical considerations.

During the study the monitor is responsible for the monitoring and reporting on the progress of the trial, for verification of data, and for source document verification. Audits before and during the study are arranged to ensure that all aspects of quality control are considered. They must be conducted either through an internal facility, but independent of the units responsible for clinical research, or through an external contractor.

The second goal of GCP is the collecting of valid study results, which has to be ensured before, during and after the study. All steps of a study including study protocol, case report forms and selection of investigators are relevant for quality of data and therefore for the quality of results. Quality control of the study is realized by investigators, monitors, data managers and biometricians. They are supervised by auditors.

The responsibilities of an investigator are ensuring progress of the trial according to protocol, correct use of medical products, correctly and completely recorded data with signed case report forms (corrections must leave the old data readable, must be dated and signed, and reasons must be given), and ensuring the blindness of the treatment. The monitor is responsible for making sure the investigator has fulfilled these responsibilities, and for the verification of data. He or she checks the data in the case report forms with source documents and submits a report after each visit. After data management has been recorded as completely as possible, and has been certified correct, the statistical analysis may be carried out. An experienced biometrician should analyse the data according to the strategy for biometric evaluation in the protocol, ensure its integrity and present it in a manner likely to facilitate the interpretation of its clinical importance, make an account of missing, unused and spurious data, and write a comprehensive biometric report.

Reports on CCTs in homoeopathy

In principle, reporting on a CCT or another study in homoeopathy is the same as in conventional medicine. However, results of studies in homoeopathy are always heavily debated and positive results should convince highly sceptical readers from conventional medicine. Therefore, reporting on a CCT in homoeopathy should be more complete, more detailed, more exhaustive, and more convincing than usual reports in conventional medicine. A report on a homoeopathic study should not leave out any point of serious criticism.

It is beyond the scope of this chapter to give a detailed outline of how to report on CCTs and other clinical studies. But the following points, known as a standard for reports on conventional clinical trials, should at least be covered by a report on a CCT in homoeopathy:

- Date of the final study protocol and how the protocol can be obtained.
- Date of admission of the first study patient and date of the latest observation of the last patient included in the evaluation.
- All positions of responsibility in the study, especially principle investigator, participating physicians, drug supplier, trustees (if any), biometrician, grants and sponsors.

- Description how randomization and masking of treatments was done, maintained and guaranteed including date and procedure of de-masking.
- Date of completion of computerized source data file and how it can be accessed.
- Description of the performance of the study, how GCP guidelines were installed, how the study was monitored and audited. Presentation of deviations from the protocol and other irregularities. Indication of withdrawals, patients lost to follow-up, and missing observations. Assessment of the quality of the study, its data and results.
- Characterization of the study patients.
- Demonstration and assessment of the comparability of treatment groups.
- Procedure of statistical analysis, how drop-outs and missing data were handled, statistical methods used.
- Answers on the matter of investigation, especially estimation of outcome variables and confirmatory hypothesis testing.
- Tolerability, safety, undesired events, and adverse therapy (drug) reactions observed.
- Further results of the study, further questions and new hypotheses.

References

Albrecht, H. and Frühwald, M. (1995) Konsensus-Konferenz der Karl und Veronica Carstens-Stiftung: Placebo in der klinischen Forschung zur Homöopathie. *Forschende Komplementärmedizin*, **2**, 36–7.

Bauer, P. and Köhne, K. (1994) Evaluation of experiments with adaptive interim analyses. *Biometrics*, **50**, 1029–41.

Bauer, P. and Röhmel, J. (1995) An adaptive method for establishing a dose–response relationship. *Statistics in Medicine*, **14**, 1595–1607.

Boissel, J.P., Collet, J.P., Moleur, P. *et al.* (1992) Surrogate endpoints: A basis for a rational approach. *European Journal of Clinical Pharmacology*, **43**, 235–44.

Brown, B.W. (1980) The cross-over experiment for clinical trials. *Biometrics*, **36**, 69–79.

Bullinger, M. (ed.) (1991) Lebensqualität bei kardiovaskulären Erkrankungen. Göttingen, Hogrefe.

CPMP Working Party on Efficacy of Medicinal Products (1991) Good Clinical Practice for Trials of Medicinal Products in the European Community. In: *Klinische Arzneimittelprüfungen in der EG*, Aulendorf, Editio Cantor, 9–33.

Deklaration von Helsinki des Weltärztebundes, Hong Kong 1989 (1991) In: *Klinische Arzneimittelprüfungen in der EG*, Aulendorf, Editio Cantor, 93–7. (See also World Medical Association Declaration.)

Ernst, E. and Resch, K.L. (1995) The 'optional cross-over design' for randomized controlled trials. *Fundamental and Clinical Pharmacology*, **9**, 508–11.

European Committee for Homoeopathy. *Homoeopathy in Europe 1994.* Appendix 1: Programme of basic teaching standards. Rotterdam.

European Committee for Homoeopathy. *Homoeopathy in Europe 1995*. Rotterdam.

Gaus, W. (1990) Design von Studien zur Wirksamkeit von Naturheilverfahren – dargestellt an einem Beispiel aus der Homöopathie und aus der Diätetik. In: H. Albrecht and G. Franz (eds): *Naturheilverfahren. Zum Stand der Forschung*. Berlin, Springer-Verlag, 129–38.

Gaus, W. (1993) Kontrollierte Studien bei niedergelassenen Ärzten: Probleme und Chancen. *Zeitschrift für Phytotherapie*, **14**, 76–82.

Gaus, W. (1994) The efficacy of classical homoeopathic therapy for chronic headaches. Biometrical report (available from the author).

Gaus, W. and Högel, J. (1995) Studies on the efficacy of unconventional therapies. Problems and designs. *Arzneimittel-Forschung/Drug Research*, **45**, 88–92.

Good Clincial Practice in the European Community (1991) German translation: Gute klinische Praxis für die klinische Prüfung von Arzneimitteln in der Europäischen Gemeinschaft. In: *Klinische Arzneimittelprüfung in der EG*. Aulendorf, Editio Cantor, 34–63. (See also CPMP.)

Good Manufacturing Practice for Pharmaceutical Products (Draft) (1992) In: 32. Report, WHO Technical Report Series 823.

Guggenmoos-Holzmann, I., Bloomfield, K., Brenner, H. and Flick, U. (1995) *Quality of life and health*. Berlin, Blackwell.

Guyatt, G., Sackett, D., Taylor, D.W. *et al.* (1986) Determining optimal therapy – randomized trials in individual patients. *New England Journal of Medicine*, **314**, 889–92.

Guyatt, G., Sackett, D., Adachi, J. *et al.* (1988) A clinician's guide for conducting randomized trials in individual patients. *Canadian Medical Association Journal*, **139**, 497–503.

Guyatt, G.H., Heyting, A., Jaeschke, R. *et al.* (1990) N of 1 randomized trials for investigating new drugs. *Controlled Clinical Trials*, **11**, 88–100.

Högel, J., Walach, H. and Gaus, W. (1994) Change-to-open-label design. Proposal and discussion of a new design for clinical parallel-group double-masked trials. *Arzneimittel Forschung/Drug Research*, **44**, 97–9.

Hulley, S.B. and Cummings, S.R. (1988) *Designing clinical research*. London, Williams and Wilkins.

Jones, B. and Lewis, J.A. (1995) The case for cross-over trials in phase III. *Statistics in Medicine*, **14**, 1025–38.

Kiene, H. (1996) A critique of the double-blind clinical trial. Part 1. *Alternative Therapies in Health and Medicine*, **2**(1), 74–80.

Kiene, H. (1996) A critique of the double-blind clinical trial. Part 2. *Alternative Therapies in Health and Medicine*, **2**(2), 59–64.

Koenig, P. and Swoboda, F. (1987) Acidum Succinicum 30x – A drug proving. *British Homoeopathic Journal*, **76**, 19–29.

Lachin, J.M. (1981) Introduction to sample size determination and power analysis for clinical trials. *Controlled Clinical Trials*, **2**, 93–113.

Lange-deKlerk, E.S.M. de, Feenstra, L., Kuik, D.J., Blommers, J. and Bezemer, P.D. (1995) Biometric problems in trials on homoeopathy. In: G. Anks, L. Edler, R. Holle, W. Köpcke, R. Lorenz and J. Windeler (eds): *Biometrie und unkonventionelle Medizin*. Band 3, Biometrische Berichte. Münster-Hiltrup, Landwirtschaftsverlag, 91–100.

Mau, J. (1993) Cross-allocation of patients to two treatments with randomization option. Forschungsbericht 93/94, Düsseldorf, Heinrich Heine Universität.

Olschewski, M. and Scheurlen, H. (1985) Comprehensive Cohort Study: an alternative to randomized consent design in a breast preservation trial. *Methods of Information in Medicine*, **24**, 131–4.

Pocock, S.J. (1983) *Clinical trials*. Chichester, Wiley.

Reilly, D.T. (1994) Certificate of Primary Care Homoeopathy (Editorial). *British Homoeopathic Journal*, **83**, 57.

Reilly, D.T. (1995) Clarifying competence by defining its limits. Lessons from the Glasgow Education Model of Homoeopathic Training. *Complementary Therapies in Medicine*, **3**, 21–4.

Reilly, D.T., Taylor, M.A., McSharry, C. and Aitchinson, T. (1986) Is homoeopathy a placebo response? Controlled trial of homoeopathic potency with pollen in hayfever as model. *The Lancet*, **II**, 881–6.

Reilly, D.T., Taylor, M.A., Beattie, N.G.M. *et al.* (1994) Is evidence for homoeopathy reproducible? *The Lancet*, **344**, 1601–6.

Reilly, D.T. and Taylor, M. (1993) Developing integrated medicine. *Complementary Therapies in Medicine*, **1** (Suppl. 1), 1–50.

Righetti, M. (1988) Forschung in der Homöopathie – Wissenschaftliche Grundlagen, Problematik und Ergebnisse. Göttingen, Ulrich Burgdorf.

Ritter, H. (1966) Ein homöotherapeutischer doppelter Blindversuch und seine Problematik. *Hippocrates*, **12**, 472–6.

Senn, S. (1993) Inherent difficulties with active control equivalence studies. *Statistics in Medicine*, **12**, 2367–75.

Senn, S. (1995) A personal view of some controversies in allocating treatment to patients in clinical trials. *Statistics in Medicine*, **14**, 2661–74.

Shipley, M., Berry, H., Broster, G., Jenkins, M., Clover, A. and Williams, I. (1983) Controlled trial of homoeopathic treatment of osteoarthritis. *The Lancet*, **I**, 97–8.

The Faculty of Homoeopathy (1995) Proposed minimum clinical standards. SIMILE 5, 10.

Walach, H. (1993) Does a highly diluted homoeopathic drug act as a placebo in healthy volunteers? Experimental study of Belladonna 30C in double-masked crossover design. *Journal of Psychosomatic Research*, **37**, 851–60.

Walach, H. (1996) Verblindung in klinischen Homöopathie-Studien? In: J. Hornung (ed.): *Forschungsmethoden in der Komplementärmedizin*. Stuttgart, Schattauer.

Walach, H., Linsemann, E. and Reisenegger, I. (1994) Wirksamkeit einer komplementärmedizinischen stationären Behandlung der atopischen Dermatitis – Ergebnisse einer katamnestischen Fragebogenstudie. *Forschende Komplementärmedizin*, **1**, 216–24.

Weiser, M. *et al.* (1994) Randomisierte plazebokontrollierte Doppelblindstudie zur Untersuchung der klinischen Wirksamkeit der homöopathischen Euphorium compositum Nasentropfen S bei chronischer Sinusitis. *Forschende Komplementärmedizin*, **1**, 251–9.

Wiesenauer, M. and Lüdtke, R. (1995) The treatment of pollinosis with Galphimia glauca D4 – a randomized placebo-controlled double-masked clinical trial. *Phytomedicine*, **2**, 3–6.

Wiesenauer, M. and Gaus, W. (1991) Wirksamkeitsnachweis eines Homöopathikums bei chronischer Polyarthritis. Eine randomizierte Doppelblindstudie bei niedergelassenen Ärzten. *Aktuelle Rheumatologie*, **16**, 1–21.

World Medical Association Declaration of Helsinki, Hong Kong 1989 (1991) In: *Klinische Arzneimittelprüfungen in der EG*. Aulendorf, Editio Cantor, 89–92. (See also Deklaration von Helsinki.)

Chapter 3

Methodology beyond controlled clinical trials

Harald Walach

Introduction

Nowadays it is a general consensus that randomized controlled trials (RCTs) which are usually carried out double blind are the gold standard of clinical trial methodology (Füllgraf, 1985; Feinstein, 1980). They are usually employed within the context of phase III studies, and designed to answer the question whether a new treatment, usually pharmacological, is superior to pure non-specific placebo treatment for a specific disease. They normally rest on a series of animal and toxicological studies, and there is usually a sound theoretic framework which links the purported causal pharmacological agent to the disease process in question. The RCT is meant to show that the novel pharmacological agent which was proven to be effective in animal models and in vitro, and which can be expected to be useful in humans due to a pharmacological theory, is also useful in clinical context. Normally, there is one pharmacological agent whose efficacy is to be evaluated with respect to one specific type of disease. By virtue of the placebo controlled methodology it is possible to answer the question whether this new pharmacological agent is causally remedial in a certain disease.

Homoeopathy, on the other hand, is not a single specific treatment for a single disease, neither is it a novel treatment, but it is a well established complex theory with many remedial substances for various types of diseases, resting on its own foundations on how to administer them. If one were to extend the analogy from conventional clinical trials to homoeopathy, then one would have to conduct as many clinical trials for as many diseases and as many remedies used in homoeopathy in order to show causal efficacy for all of them. This clearly is an impossible task. The call for RCTs in the framework of homoeopathic research therefore seems to be more of a global demand to show causal therapeutic efficacy. The question, then, is not whether a certain type of pharmacological agent is remedially causal in treating a specific disease, but rather, whether a therapeutic approach as a whole, such as homoeopathy, can be regarded as causally and specifically active in general.

In order to provide an answer to this complex question, I propose to disentangle it and to divide it into separate sub-questions. They divide into four sub-questions which will be treated separately:

1. General clinical effectiveness.
2. Comparative clinical efficacy.

3 Efficacy compared to proven gold standard or standard therapy.
4 Genuine causal efficacy of homoeopathic remedies.

General clinical effectiveness

The foremost question to answer is: how effective is homoeopathy as normally practised in general clinical practice for what type of diseases in what kind of patients? As yet, there is only limited evidence as to whether homoeopathic therapy is effective, and in what type of diseases, and to what extent. Some retrospective audit studies have been published in the past (Haidvogl, Lehner and Resch, 1993; Diemer, Meili and de Pedroni, 1991; Blackstone, 1994; Castellsagu, 1992; Pöllmann and Hildebrandt, 1985; Queralt Gimeno, 1991; Rastogi *et al.*,1993; Van Berckel Smit, 1993; Van Haselen and Fisher, 1992, 1994; Zeeden, 1995; Rückert, 1854; van Erp and Brands, 1996; Gerhard, 1996; Gerhard, Keller and Monga, 1995, 1996; Eizayaga and Eizayaga, 1996), but to my knowledge no large scale prospective studies have been conducted documenting clinical effects of homoeopathic therapy. There is one large scale documentation study ongoing (Walach *et al.,* 1996) and some more studies are under way. The only evidence we have up to now whether homoeopathic therapy is effective, is the history of homoeopathy which indirectly proves that it does seem to produce some positive outcome for some patients, although we know that there have been a lot of therapies which initially in uncontrolled settings were found to be quite effective but could not be proven to be superior to placebo treatment when submitted to controlled clinical trials (Roberts, 1993). This, however, does not invalidate that these therapies were in some way effective for treating the disease in question, albeit not for the alleged reasons, which were founded on some fallacious therapeutic theory. On the other hand, there have been other therapeutic systems which have been invented at the same time as homoeopathy, e.g. Brownianism, which did not survive the test of history (Schwanitz, 1983). There apparently are no other examples of only historically validated therapies with doubtful experimental evidence apart from homoeopathy, which are still to some extent important for their practical implications. There seems to be some therapeutic efficacy in homoeopathy which helped homoeopathy survive many impugnments by the medical establishment. Had it not been for the many attested positive results which people experienced by homoeopathic therapy, it would not have been possible for homoeopathy to survive alongside the development of potent pharmaceutical agents in conventional medicine. However, we still do not know to what extent homoeopathic therapy really is effective in ordinary practice. The documentation of this baseline healing rate would be valuable evidence.

Comparative clinical evidence – experimental or quasi-experimental control?

In order to see whether this baseline homoeopathic healing rate or effectiveness is superior to what we know from conventional medical treatment it is necessary to have comparative studies. We could conduct simultaneously two documentation studies, one documenting patients under homoeopathic treatment, and another one documenting patients under conventional treatment, without a randomization procedure, but in a natural setting. Thereby, a quasi-experimental control group can be established which by appropriate matching procedures would yield valuable comparative data. Usually it is thought that randomization is superior to any type of quasi-experimental control. This is certainly true from a purely biometrical or methodological vantage point. For randomization guarantees relatively comparable treatment groups, because chance allocation of persons to groups distributes possibly confounding variables equally over both groups, whereas comparison of naturally selected groups always introduces possibly confounding factors and thereby distorts the outcome measure, which in turn hampers internal validity (Rossi, Freeman and Hoffmann, 1988).

On the other hand, randomization is an invasive procedure which when applied properly together with informed consent, yields highly selective samples of patients (Howard, Cox and Saunders, 1990). It has been shown that the same substance, Naproxen in cancer pain patients, had totally different effects when given under the conditions of blinded study design with informed consent, or unwittingly, compared with placebo (Bergmann *et al.*, 1994). In this particular study, Naproxen applied clinically without the specific ramifications of an RCT was less effective than placebo within an RCT. This shows that results gleaned from controlled trials can by no means be transferred literally to clinical situations.

Apart from psychological expectations and attitudes, created within the framework of an RCT, which can not be controlled, there is the problem of attrition and loss to follow-up, which is a common research problem, but more so for randomized trials. Since patients are not free to choose a treatment within an RCT, and since doctors on the other hand seek to enrol as many patients as possible, patients are likely either not to enter the trial, or, if enrolled, to draw back. In the case of the large Antabuse trial in the USA, this led to the problem that less than 9 per cent of the possible target population was treated within the trial and the results, although internally valid, were worthless for practical purposes (Howard, Cox and Saunders, 1990). This suggests that randomization is itself a highly problematic procedure because it also compromises internal validity: 'Randomization has been transformed from a method that was intended to assist scientific investigation to a dogma by which research is reflexively judged. We would argue for the opposite stance – randomization should always be explicitly justified. An investigator must explain why randomization was undertaken, the extent to which it was successfully implemented, and whether this strategy compensated for the accompanying loss of generalizability.' (p. 75).

Many patients, especially those in complementary treatment, are not willing to be randomized into any type of treatment, and usually they have strong preferences for complementary treatment, because this is what they chose to have, and because they have usually had experience with conventional medicine (Furnham and Forey, 1994; Furnham and Bhagrath, 1993; Furnham and Smith, 1988; Furnham, 1992; Furnham, Vincent and Wood, 1995). It might well be the case that homoeopathic treatment shows its effectiveness only when patient co-operation is unrestricted. As the homoeopathic doctor has to rely on very specific and often highly intimate types of information which can only be gleaned from the patient when there is a full trusting relationship, it could be that the homoeopathic treatment is not fully effective when there is not full consensus about the treatment. Therefore, it seems to be worthwhile to take into account the methodological shortcomings of quasi-experimental control and to opt for a better external validity which is usually higher in a quasi-experimental setting (Smith, 1980; Chen and Rossi, 1983; Rossi and Freeman, 1982; Cronbach, 1982).

Such a type of study would be able to show whether homoeopathic treatment is comparable in ordinary clinical setting to that of conventional medical treatment for the specific types of patients who choose to either have this or the other treatment. It could be argued that we then never know whether this would be true for all sorts of patients, or only for those who have for some reason or other chosen homoeopathy. But then, this question is quite academic indeed. For it is the particular patients in real life, who choose homoeopathy as it is, who either have or have no success and who either reduce or increase the cost of health care.

Randomized comparisons

In order to find out whether a homoeopathic approach is comparable or superior to a standard treatment in general and for all sorts of patients, a randomized comparison study would be appropriate. This type of study could be conducted in a two or three legged design. In a two legged study patients suffering from a specific type of disease are being randomized to receive either conventional standard treatment or homoeopathic treatment. No attempt will be made to blind the treatment. This type of study could supplement the quasi-experimental approach in order to answer the question whether homoeopathic treatment is equal or superior to conventional treatment.

In order to find out whether the homoeopathic case taking or the homoeopathic prescription is the decisive point in question, a third study leg could be introduced. Patients in this group could receive a homoeopathic case taking interview but will afterwards be randomized to receive conventional treatment. By comparing homoeopathic treatment alone against conventional treatment alone against homoeopathic case taking plus conventional treatment, the effects of the joint effects of homoeopathic case taking plus homoeopathic remedy could be somewhat disentangled and estimated by the interaction effect, to speak in the language of analysis of variance. This is certainly possible only in cases where the conventional treatment has a known efficacy. Since blinding is not applied, homoeopathic treatment is in no way hampered. But because randomization is introduced, one has to reckon with the problem that patients might be randomized into the homoeopathic treatment group, who are not prepared – in the fullest sense of the word – to open themselves in a way necessary for the homoeopathic doctor to receive the full information needed for a successful prescription. It has not been investigated so far whether there is a difference in treatment between patients who have selected homoeopathic treatment themselves and patients who have been allotted such a treatment. It seems necessary that before setting out for randomized comparison studies this question should be addressed in preliminary studies which compare baseline healing rates for patients who have selected homoeopathy themselves and patients who have been allotted this type of treatment.

Double-blind randomized clinical trials

The question to be answered by a double-blind randomized controlled clinical trial with placebo control is whether the homoeopathic remedies as such are superior to placebo treatment. This amounts to the question whether homoeopathic remedies are causal for the therapeutic progress. It could well be the case that in the long run it is difficult or even impossible to establish the causal efficacy of homoeopathic remedies over and against placebo. This would lead to the conclusion that homoeopathic therapy is a placebo effect. But what would be the conclusion if studies of types 1 to 3 (documentation, clinical comparison, randomized comparison) should prove that homoeopathic therapy can be quite effective and can be as effective as conventional treatment? If it should be the case that homoeopathic treatment proves effective in a clinical sense but not causally superior in placebo controlled studies would this mean that homoeopathic therapy is not effective? We then obviously would have to conclude that homoeopathic therapy can be a powerful therapeutic tool although we would at the same time know that homoeopathic remedies as such are not causal for the therapeutic progress. For it could be the case that the whole ritual of homoeopathic case taking, treatment, consulting, and remedy prescription are powerful therapeutic agents and the homoeopathic remedy would be only a kind of vehicle to convey the therapeutic effort of the doctor and to initiate the self-healing capacity of the patient.

In the light of so many proven pharmaceutical approaches which, from the clinical point of view, are only moderately effective, this still would be valuable evidence as to the general therapeutic potency of homoeopathy. Maybe the result of such a staged effort of studying homoeopathic therapy would be that there is no proof of causal agency of homoeopathic remedies, but of general clinical efficacy of homoeopathic therapy. This then would mean that homoeopathy is an effective therapy although the causal agency of homoeopathic remedies is negligible. This certainly would be a bewildering result but certainly not one which denies general effectiveness to homoeopathic therapy. I would like to warn against the short cut conclusion that either homoeopathic therapy relies on causally efficacious agency of homoeopathic remedies or else it has to be abandoned as quackery.

Let me take the case of psychotherapy as an example. There are many studies which have proven beyond doubt that psychotherapy is superior to no therapy or to therapy which is only marginally psychotherapeutic (Grawe, Donati and Bernauer, 1994). And yet it has not been proven and is highly difficult to prove that ingredients of psychotherapy are causal agents for the disease processes in question (Frank and Kupfer, 1992). There is a broad discussion within psychotherapy research about common factors of therapy which are common to many therapeutic approaches and which are not causally specific but genuine to many interventions (Stricker and Gold,

1993). Still nobody would say that psychotherapy is quackery. On the other hand, there are many examples of pharmacological potent and causal agents which are proven by randomized double-blind clinical studies and which in clinical context reveal not much of therapeutic effectiveness on the whole. For example in rheumatology a case can be made that there are potent analgesics, anti-inflammatory and disease-modifying agents which are proven to be effective in clinical studies but which do not live up to their expectations in long-term clinical management (Gabriel and Bombardier, 1989; Arnold *et al.*, 1990; Capell *et al.*, 1990; Paulus *et al.*, 1990; Pullar and Capell, 1985). In migraine, prophylactic beta-blocking agents and calcium-antagonists have been proven to be effective in many patients. And still, there is a substantial percentage of patients who do not gain any profit from these pharmaceuticals. In many medical disciplines there is a large knowledge gap between what we know from randomized trials about the effectiveness of pharmacological active agents and long-term clinical management in daily practice (Füllgraf, 1985; Charlton, 1991).

Perhaps the time is ripe now to broaden our view and to see causal efficacy of pharmacological agents as only one maybe necessary but not sufficient condition for the clinical management of patients. Maybe it is time to acknowledge that it is not only causal efficacy but general clinical effectiveness which should be sought for. In that sense it could well be true that homoeopathy is a truly complementary type of therapy, namely one whose pharmacological efficacy might be minimal, but whose general clinical efficacy is good enough to warrant it a status as a good clinical approach to many diseases. But in order to achieve this, it is not enough and sufficient to just study the causal efficacy of homoeopathic remedies in double-blind placebo controlled studies but to envisage the whole broad spectrum of clinical effects.

Problems of RCTs specific to homoeopathy trials

Surely this statement must not be taken as a subtle withdrawal from generally accepted methodological standard, common sense and agreement. But it should be taken as a warning against solely relying on double-blind randomized methodology to study the question of efficacy of homoeopathy. I have argued that the question of effectiveness is best disentangled into the questions of general effectiveness or baseline healing rates, of comparative effectiveness in natural and randomized settings, and of causal efficacy. Whereas the study of causal efficacy via RCTs is straightforward within the medical scientific community, it is less so within the context of homoeopathic research. I have hinted at the problems which generally beset RCTs and which are common to any approach, since they are inherent in the methodology, namely the problems of selectivity, attrition and lack of representivity. There is another problem of this methodology when it comes to evaluating homoeopathy: the problem of insecurity engendered in the treating physicians, which I have elaborated on elsewhere (Walach, 1996). The argument is now outlined.

Normally, RCTs test one treatment regime against placebo. At the most, there are one or two alternative regimens, if the treatment modality fails, or else there are dose-increasing or reducing regimens, when side-effects occur or the treatment lacks effectiveness. But in any case, there is a fairly restricted range of actions to be taken in account by the study physician within the context of a traditional RCT. The information necessary to take the corresponding steps are usually given at the outset. The situation is different in the case of evaluating homoeopathy: since the treatment within homoeopathy is dependent on both the fact that the *decisive* information is gleaned – the so called totality of symptoms, i.e. the totality of *relevant* symptoms – and the course of the treatment, the course of action to be taken is not fixed at the outset of an RCT of homoeopathy.

While during the course of a normal, non-blind treatment of homoeopathy there is always the question whether the choice of the remedy was correct and thus a considerable insecurity is normal, in a blinded treatment this generic insecurity is superseded by the insecurity of whether a failure in a patient to react to the treatment is due to the wrong choice of the remedy or to the fact that the patient has been randomized into the placebo group (leaving out of consideration, for the present purpose, the equally likely alternative that homoeopathy is a fake; but this certainly would not be generating insecurity in a professed homoeopathic doctor in the context of an RCT). Thus, a homoeopathic doctor within the context of a blinded RCT has to decide whether a lack of positive reaction in a patient is likely to be due to the wrong choice of remedy or to placebo-allocation. This, however, means that the doctor is making an attribution judgement, whose nature and impact cannot be at all controlled.

It was precisely because attributions are so powerful that the blinded RCT came to be employed in the evaluation of drugs. Now we have to face the disturbing fact that this very same methodology, introduced to control for attribution processes, engenders a new species of uncontrollable attributions: the attribution of intermediate treatment outcome in the patient to a subjectively evaluated likelihood of group allocation. This attribution, I contend, could have profound impacts on the *internal* validity of such a trial: if a doctor has a tendency to wrongly attribute therapy-failures to the administration of placebos, he will under-treat his patients, thereby minimizing placebo effects. If he has the opposite tendency, he will over-treat his patients, thereby maximizing placebo effects. Since it is likely that treatment failures occur across groups and the doctor in a blinded trial has no means of deciding the group allocation of his patients, he will produce false positives and false negatives, depending on his personal attribution style, both of which reduce the 'true' difference between groups. For if a patient randomized into the treatment group shows no clearcut effect after the first prescription, because the choice of the remedy was wrong (according to homoeopathic theory), but the doctor decides that the failure is likely due to his patient having received placebo, he will not invest enough energy in finding the correct symptoms and thereby produce a false negative outcome. If, on the other hand, a patient randomized into the placebo group shows an unclear picture and the doctor decides that this must be due to a wrong choice of remedy, he will try harder to find the surmised symptoms thereby overtreating the patient and possibly producing a false positive outcome. Because we do not know how such attribution processes work in complex situations, and because it is highly likely that such effects are idiosyncratic, they cannot be controlled for. Such processes clearly hamper the internal validity of a blinded RCT of homoeopathy.

Another factor should be considered: homoeopathy relies heavily on the acquisition of relevant symptomatic details from the patient by the doctor. Sometimes these relevant details can be of quite an intimate nature, e.g. if the central symptoms pertain to sexuality, or personal psychological habits, like jealousy, or central life experiences, such as a past trauma. It is obvious that patient and doctor likewise need the protection of a secure therapeutic relationship, in order to deal with such material. In a controlled trial this relationship is beset with the problem of insecurity, which in subtle ways might alter the performance of the doctor or the willingness of the patient to share important information. If this should indeed be the case this would be a factor which hampers internal validity of such trials.

Since it is unknown to what extent such problems do indeed occur – I have only conducted thought experiments on these questions and no empirical data are known – it would be wise and necessary to investigate these questions first, before the purported internal validity of blinded RCTs is extrapolated to research in homoeopathy.

Provings

A genuine trait of homoeopathy is the reliance on the law of similars, which states that the remedies have to be applied such that the state of symptoms presented by a patient has to be matched to the symptoms which are being produced by the remedy in healthy volunteers. This is the question of homoeopathic remedy proving; more concretely, whether the symptoms produced by homoeopathic remedies in volunteers are different from placebo symptoms. There is little evidence as yet that the symptoms of the homoeopathic remedies are different from placebo symptoms (Walach, 1993, 1994, 1996; Dantas *et al.* 1997). It would be a totally different strand of investigation to study this question. On the one hand, there are mostly qualitative results of proving studies which seem to have produced the varied and different symptom pictures in homoeopathic materia medica, and which have proved to be valuable in clinical practice. On the other hand, little attempts have been made to validate this claim in experimentally controlled studies. One way to do this would be to qualitatively gather the symptoms of these volunteers in carefully blinded experimental protocols, to translate the symptoms into repertory language, to add up remedy specific symptoms, and thereby convert them into quantitative scores, comparing the remedy scores in the experimental group to the scores in a placebo group. This would answer the question whether the symptoms produced by homoeopathic remedies are different from placebo symptoms.

It could well be the case that this type of study would not show remedy symptoms to be different from placebo symptoms. What would this mean for homoeopathic theory? It would mean that a large part of the symptoms gathered in homoeopathic materia medica could be incidental placebo symptoms which nevertheless have contributed to a somewhat arbitrary remedy picture, which subsequently has been effectively used for treating patients. It may be the case that the pure conviction of homoeopathic practitioners that these symptoms belong to a remedy and thus make up the genuine remedy picture is enough to be used for treatment purposes. This would mean that it is the homoeopathic tradition and the homoeopathic way of gathering information which produces a healing system based maybe solely on the meaning engendered by the process and the conviction of the practitioner which nevertheless might be able to produce cures in patients. From a purely pragmatic point of view this would be enough. It would not be a proof for causal efficacy, it would not be a proof for a difference between homoeopathic remedies and placebo, but it would still not invalidate the fact that the homoeopathic therapeutic ritual as such can be a therapeutic process.

Maybe we have to rethink the notion of what it is to be therapeutic, and to what extent we need causal agents in order to be therapeutic. It is an often unspoken implicit and sometimes outspoken tenet that only causal therapeutic agents which are causal with respect to a certain therapeutic theory can be deemed to be truly effective (Grünbaum, 1986, 1989). And this certainly is the prevalent scientific point of view. But it is already some years ago that Frank (1981, 1987, 1989) advocated that even the purely causal theories of medicine are only one way to achieve a therapeutic ritual which in the end enhances personal self-efficacy and thus contributes to healing in the patient. Maybe there are many types of therapeutic rituals which can do the same, and the causal agents deemed necessary by orthodox medical teaching are only one way of achieving a potent therapeutic ritual. Maybe homoeopathy has succeeded in establishing a therapeutic ritual on its own which is nevertheless therapeutically very efficient and potent, without employing a causal agent. It might well be the case that it is necessary for homoeopaths to believe that they are dealing with causal agents by employing homoeopathic remedies. But it could also be the case that this claim is wrong, and it is enough to have the belief in such a causal agent in order to enact a potent therapeutic ritual which allows the patient to harness his or her self-healing powers.

Therefore, we should adopt a broad framework for studying homoeopathy, one which starts from the general clinical effectiveness and asks the question of causal efficacy of homoeopathic remedies only at the very end. Answering this question in the negative says only as much that the effective principle in homoeopathic therapy is or is not causal in the ordinary sense of the word. It does not say that homoeopathic therapy is not effective. And it is doubtful whether pharmacological causal agency is the only and best way to achieve therapeutic efficacy. It might well be the case that it is the whole therapeutic ritual including the belief of the practitioner, the belief of the patient and a therapeutic rationale, which is convincing to both of them, that fosters cures in patients.

References

Arnold, M.H., O'Callaghan, J., McCredie, M., Beller, E.M., Kelly, B. and Brooks, R.H. (1990) Comparative controlled trial of low-dose weekly methotrexate versus azathioprine in rheumatoid arthritis: 3-year prospective study. *British Journal of Rheumatology,* **29**, 120–25.

Bergmann, J.-F., Chassany, O., Gandiol, J., Deblos, P., Kanis, J.A. *et al.* (1994) A randomized clinical trial of the effect of informed consent on the analgesic activity of placebo and naproxen in cancer patients. *Clinical Trials and Meta-Analysis,* **29**, 41–7.

Blackstone, V. (1994) An audit of prescribing Natrum muriaticum. *British Homoeopathic Journal,* **83**,14–19.

Capell, H.A., Marabani, M., Madhok, R., Torley, H. and Hunter, J.A. (1990) Degree and extent of response to sulphasalazine or penicillamine therapy for rheumatoid arthritis: Results from a routine clinical environment over a two-year period. *Quarterly Journal of Medicine, New Series,* **75**, 335–44.

Castellsagu, A.P.I. (1992) Evolution of 26 cases of bronchial asthma with homoeopathic treatment. *British Homoeopathic Journal,* **81**, 168–72.

Charlton, B.G. (1991) Medical practice and the double-blind, randomized controlled trial. *British Journal of General Practice,* **41,** 355–6.

Chen, H.T. and Rossi, P.H. (1983) Evaluating with sense. The theory-driven approach. *Evaluation Review,* **7**, 283–302.

Cronbach, L.J. (1982) *Designing Evaluations of Educational and Social Programs.* San Francisco: Bass.

Dantas, F., Fisher, P., Walach, H., Wieland, F., Poitevin, B. *et al.* (1997) Homoeopathic remedy provings. An international review. *British Homoeopathic Journal,* (in press).

Diemer, I., Meili, W.A. and de Pedroni (1991) Tätigkeitsbericht 1988/1989. *Deutsches Journal für Homöopathie,* **10,** 335–9.

Eizayaga, F.X. and Eizayaga, J. (1996) Homoeopathic treatment of bronchial asthma. Retrospective study of 62 cases. *British Homoeopathic Journal,* **85**, 28–33 (Abstract).

Feinstein, A. (1980) Should placebo-controlled trials be abolished? *European Journal of Clinical Pharmacology,* **17**, 1–4.

Frank, J.D. (1981) *Die Heiler: Wirkungsweisen psychotherapeutischer Beeinflussung; vom Schamanismus bis zu den modernen Therapien.* Stuttgart: Klett-Cotta.

Frank, J.D. (1987) Therapeutic components shared by all psychotherapies. In: Harvey and Parks, eds. *Psychotherapy Research and Behavior Change,* 73–122.

Frank, J.D. (1989) Non-specific aspects of treatment: the view of a psychotherapist. In: M. Shepherd and N. Sartorius, eds. *Non-Specific Aspects of Treatment.* Berne: Huber, 95–114.

Frank, E. and Kupfer, D.J. (1992) Does a placebo tablet affect psychotherapeutic treatment outcome? Results from the Pittsburgh study of maintenance therapies in recurrent depression. *Psychotherapy Research,* **2**, 102–11 (Abstract).

Füllgraf, G. (1985) Der kontrollierte klinische Versuch – Eine kritische Würdigung. *Pharmazeutische Zeitung,* **130 (51/52)**, 3309–13.

Furnham, A. (1992) Why people choose complementary medicine. *Yearbook of Cross-Cultural Medicine and Psychotherapy,* 165–96.

Furnham, A. and Bhagrath, R. (1993) A comparison of health beliefs and behaviours of clients of orthodox and complementary medicine. *British Journal of Clinical Psychology,* **32**, 237–46.

Furnham, A. and Forey, J. (1994) The attitudes, behaviors and beliefs of patients of conventional vs. complementary (alternative) medicine. *Journal of Clinical Psychology,* **50 (3)**, 458–69.

Furnham, A. and Smith C. (1988) Choosing alternative medicine: a comparison of the beliefs of patients visiting a general practitioner and a homoeopath. *Soc. Sci. Med.,* **26**, 685–9.

Furnham, A., Vincent, C. and Wood, R. (1995) The health beliefs and behaviors of three groups of complementary medicine and a general practice group of patients. *Journal of Alternative and Complementary Medicine,* **1**, 347–59 (Abstract).

Gabriel, S.E. and Bombardier, C. (1989) Clinical trials in fibrositis: a critical review and future directions. *Journal of Rheumatology,* **16 supp. 19**, 177–9.

Gerhard, I. (1996) Die Ambulanz für Naturheilkunde der Universitäts-Fauenklinik Heidelberg. In: H. Albrecht and M. Frühwald, eds. *Jahrbuch der Karl und Veronica Carstens-Stiftung.* Stuttgart: Hippokrates, 3–12.

Gerhard, I., Keller, C. and Monga, B. (1995) Homöopathische Behandlung bei weiblicher Unfruchtbarkeit. *Erfahrungsheilkunde,* **44**, 545–55 (Abstract).

Gerhard, I., Keller, C. and Monga, B. (1996) Homöopathische Behandlung bei weiblicher Unfruchtbarkeit. In: H. Albrecht and M. Frühwald, eds. *Jahrbuch der Karl und Veronica Carstens-Stiftung*. Stuttgart: Hippokrates, 217–39.

Grawe, K., Donati, R. and Bernauer, F. (1994) *Psychotherapie im Wandel. Von der Konfession zur Profession*. Göttingen: Hogrefe.

Grünbaum, A. (1986) The placebo effect in medicine and psychiatry. *Psychological Medicine,* **16**, 19–38.

Grünbaum, A. (1989) The placebo concept in medicine and psychiatry. In: M. Shepherd and N. Sartorius, eds. *Non-Specific Aspects of Treatment*. Berne: Huber, 7–38.

Haidvogl, M., Lehner, E. and Resch, D.M. (1993) Homoeopathic treatment of handicapped children. *British Homoeopathic Journal,* **82**, 227–36.

Howard, K.I., Cox, W.M. and Saunders, S.M. (1990) Attrition in substance abuse comparative treatment research: The illusion of randomization. In: L.S. Onken and J.D. Blaine, eds. *Psychotherapy and Counseling in the Treatment of Drug Abuse*. Rockville: National Institute of Drug Abuse, 66–79.

Paulus, H.E., Egger, M.J., Ward, J.R., Williams, H.J. *et al.* (1990) Analysis of improvement in individual rheumatoid arthritis patients treated with disease-modifying antirheumatic drugs, based on the findings in patients treated with placebo. *Arthritis and Rheumatism,* **33**, 477–84.

Pöllmann, L. and Hildebrandt, G. (1985) Zur Gabe von Arnica, Planta tota D3, bei kieferchirurgischen Eingriffen. *Erfahrungsheilkund,* **34**, 503–6.

Pullar, T. and Capell, H.A. (1985) A rheumatological dilemma: is it possible to modify the course of rheumatoid arthritis? Can we answer the question? *Annals of Rheumatic Diseases,* **44**, 134–40.

Queralt Gimeno, M.L. (1991) Homoeopathic treatment of ovarian cysts. *British Homoeopathic Journal,* **80**, 143–8.

Rastogi, D.P., Singh, V.P., Singh, V. and Dey, S.K. (1993) Evaluation of homoeopathic therapy in 129 asymptomatic HIV carriers. *British Homoeopathic Journal,* **82**, 4–8.

Roberts, A.H. (1993) The power of nonspecific effects in healing: implications for psychosocial and biological treatments. *Clinical Psychology Review,* **13**, 375–91.

Rossi, P.H. and Freeman, H.E. (1982) *Evaluation. A Systematic Approach* (2nd ed.). Beverly Hills: Sage.

Rossi, P.H., Freeman, H.E. and Hoffmann, G. (1988) *Programm-Evaluation. Einführung in die Methoden angewandter Sozialforschung*. Stuttgart: Enke.

Rückert, T.J. (1854) *Klinische Erfahrungen in der Homöopathie. Eine vollständige Sammlung aller, in der deutschen und ins Deutsche übertragenen homöopathischen Literatur niedergelegten Heilungen und praktischen Bemerkungen vom Jahre 1822–1850*. Leipzig: Eduard Haynel.

Schwanitz, H.J. (1983) *Homöopathie und Brownianismus 1795–1844*. Stuttgart, New York: Gustav-Fischer-Verlag.

Smith, N.L. (1980) The feasibility and desirability of experimental methods in evaluation. *Evaluation and Program Planning,* **3**, 251–6.

Stricker, Q. and Gold, J.R. (eds) (1993) *Comprehensive Handbook of Psychotherapy Integration*. New York: Plenum.

Van Berckel Smit, J.A.C.M. (1993) A pilot study evaluating the efficacy of homoeopathy in daily practice. *British Medical Journal,* **82**, 9–15.

van Erp, V.M.A. and Brands, M. (1996) Homoeopathic treatment of malaria in Ghana. *British Homoeopathic Journal,* **85**, 66–70 (Abstract).

Van Haselen, R.A. and Fisher, P. (1992) Towards a new method for improving clinical homoeopathy. *British Homoeopathic Journal,* **81,** 120–26.

Van Haselen, R. and Fisher, P. (1994) Describing and improving homoeopathy. *British Homoeopathic Journal,* **83**, 135–41.

Walach, H., Brednich, A., Heinrich, S. and Esser, P. (1996) Das Erprobungsverfahren der Innungskrankenkassen zu Homöopathie und Akupunktur. Evaluationskonzept und erste Erfahrungen. *Forschende Komplementärmedizin,* **3**, 12–20.

Walach, H. (1993) Does a highly diluted homoeopathic drug act as a placebo in healthy volunteers? *Journal of Psychosomatic Research,* **37**, 851–60.

Walach, H. (1994) Provings: the method and its future. *British Homoeopathic Journal,* **83**, 129–31.

Walach, H. (1996) Verblindung in klinischen Homöopathie-Studien? In: J. Hornung, ed. *Forschungsmethoden in der Komplementärmedizin. Über die Notwendigkeit einer methodologischen Erneuerung*. Stuttgart: Schattauer, 1–16.

Zeeden, H. (1995) Einsatz von Einzelmitteln an der Kurklinik Benediktusquelle vom 01.02.91 bis 20.09.92. *Allgemeine Homöopathische Zeitung,* **1**, 19–27.

Part II

Homoeopathic Provings

Chapter 4

The role of drug provings in the homoeopathic concept

Frank Wieland

Introduction

In his book *Principles and Practice of Homoeopathy* M.L. Dhawale has stated that: 'He who does not know what he seeketh, will not understand what he findeth'.

This chapter will try to demonstrate what the proving doctor is seeking when he or she performs a homoeopathic drug proving and what is necessary for the proper understanding and evaluation of the results. First, it is necessary to define what is meant by the term 'homoeopathic concept' in the title. It refers to the concept of applying a single remedy for a given totality of symptoms, according to the law of similars.

From drug provings we obtain a drug picture, which is then related to the patient, taking into account all the presenting symptoms.

Aim of Provings: the role of the proving doctor

The purpose of homoeopathic drug provings is to seek the innate character of a remedy, which is more an aspect of quality rather than quantity. A proving is not undertaken in order to prove the effect of a drug, but rather to test its qualities.

In allopathic medicine the main goal of provings is to provide evidence of a predetermined effect, i.e. reduction of blood pressure or anxiety, etc. The effect is measured by statistical methods and is usually related to placebo or an established therapy. For homoeopathic drug provings the approach is fundamentally different. The concept of homoeopathy assumes that the remedy, if given to a healthy person, affects the vital force of the whole organism and that the alterations of the vital force are shown by individual symptoms in the mind, intellect and body of the volunteer (Wieland, 1996).

The range of enquiry is not a predetermined field; all symptoms of mind, intellect and body are registered and documented. Kent says in his lectures: 'the best way to study a (homoeopathic) remedy is to make a proving of it.' This is obviously correct, for the homoeopathic physician it is essential to have personal experience of drug provings (Hahnemann, 1986) because the similarity of the proving symptoms to the illness of the patient gives an understanding of what, for example, a burning headache is or permits the experience of the psychological symptoms of Hepar sulphuris Calcareum: 'The slightest cause irritates him and makes him extremely vehement' (Hering, 1971).

The author himself had an experience when he made a proving with Hepar sulphuris which helped him to understand a symptom described by a patient. Before the proving he had more or less dismissed the patient's complaint as an attempt to find an excuse for a violent nature. However, after having taken three globules of Hepar sulphuris C30 3–4 times a day for two days, the author himself experienced a strong desire to hit people for no valid reason: perhaps when standing in a crowded bus, or when someone accidentally brushed against him. He had not experienced these sudden and violent impulses before and they were difficult to control.

By undertaking the proving, he went into a state of suffering similar to that of the patient. This meant he could experience a remarkable change in his own emotional state, which led him to a much deeper understanding of the patient's problem.

But in order to be aware that changes are taking place, it is necessary to know what the status of the patient was before the proving. For volunteers taking part in a homoeopathic drug proving, this is achieved by the taking of a history of prior symptoms, illnesses, and the current state of mind and health before the proving begins.

Taking a Case History

For the proving doctor, the taking of a thorough case history before the pre-observation period of the proving is mandatory for the following reasons, which are mentioned in Section 2 of the Minimum Standard for Homoeopathic Drug Provings launched by the ECH Sub committee on Drug Provings (see Appendix):

Case taking is obligatory:

- for safety; to ensure that the volunteer is healthy enough to take part in a proving
- to give a baseline of actual state of health and symptoms
- to ensure that the volunteer has properly understood the purpose and procedure of the proving, is reliable (§126, *Organon*), and is able to explain any symptoms precisely enough.

It is a difficult process to judge which symptoms of a proving belong to the remedy, which to the patient or which possibly to the placebo effect. The personal experience of the proving doctor is essential for developing the art of conducting provings. This may be one reason why provings are currently performed in so many different ways. In addition, provings have many different purposes. The manufacturers of homoeopathic remedies in some cases perform provings for legal reasons, to justify the use of the substance by showing that it has an effect. To a certain degree the designs for both types of provings may be the same, but if we wish to do a proving for the sake of deriving the remedy out of the symptoms, case taking is mandatory, for the reasons given earlier.

David Riley from Santa Fe, New Mexico, who has carried out approximately 50 provings for different pharmaceutical firms (Riley, 1996) spends on average two hours with each volunteer before beginning the proving. He does not, however, perform a classical homoeopathic case taking but does go through an 8-page evaluation form with the volunteers. The author feels obliged to stress that the most essential prerequisite for a good homoeopathic drug proving is a thorough case taking. He would also like to stress how rewarding it is to perform provings and how poor the current research methodology appears to be.

It is clear, therefore, that a really good proving requires a large amount of time and thought. It should be the aim of all those involved in provings to establish a system of worldwide co-operation and exchange of data, so that all homoeopaths can benefit from the exchange of knowledge.

It is necessary to promote the importance of case history taking, because it is often not understood that a good case history taking 'prepares the occurrence of symptoms'. 'During the course of a successful clinical interview a happy relationship develops between the two (patient and doctor)' (Dhawale, 1985).

The aim of a proving is to recognize the nature, the innate character of a remedy. This nature can best be recognized by carefully eliciting the impressions and feelings that the patient is experiencing whilst under the influence of the remedy. Often there are no symptoms reported; sometimes because they are so subtle that the volunteer does not mention them. Only a very close and trusting relationship between proving doctor and volunteer (which J.P. Jansen once called 'the heart to heart contact') will bring those symptoms to light (Jansen, 1995).

Proving of remedies is both an art and a science (Nagpaul, 1987). When it is reduced merely to a science, the symptoms brought to light by the art are lost.

The Five Steps of Hering

Many discussions about how to carry out provings have dealt with the question of the most suitable design and on how to decide whether the symptom has occurred as a result of the action of the remedy or the placebo. The placebo question is not discussed in depth in this chapter; suffice it to say that even if placebo symptoms should occur during a proving this is not ultimately important for the decision on whether or not a symptom belongs to the remedy picture. This is because when a symptom occurs in a proving there is first a certain **probability** that it belongs to the remedy picture as Hering describes in the Preface of Vol. 1 *Guiding Symptoms* (Hering, 1974).

The second step, **confirmation**, is obtained when the same symptoms are experienced by several volunteers during the same proving, or when they recur in other provings. It is very interesting that the same symptoms have been observed when provings with the same remedy have been conducted with different designs, regardless of whether this is with or without placebo (Bayr, 1983; Mezger, 1970). Besides confirming the symptoms by comparing them with other provings, there is another possibility mentioned in the third step of Hering – **corroboration**, which means to look for physiological or pathological effects of the drug when taken in a raw substance, i.e. by accident (Belladonna fruits taken by children) or in daily life (onions – Cepa allium; cigarettes – tabacum).

But the question of whether or not a symptom which has been found in a proving is a reliable symptom for the application of the remedy finds its answer in Hering's fourth step: **verification**. The drug is given to the sick according to the symptoms it has produced in the healthy and the cures made are the verifications. When this has been done by numerous therapists with success, it finally leads to Hering's fifth step, **characteristics**. When a symptom is consistently verified by the cures it becomes characteristic for the remedy. How many times and in which way the cure has to be documented is still open to discussion. Solving this question is one of the aims for the future.

This chapter is a very brief survey of the science and art of provings. During the last few years there have been numerous activities relating to drug provings all around the world, one of which is presented here.

The ECH Sub committee on Drug Provings (European Committee for Homoeopathy, 1994) has made considerable efforts in Europe to promote drug provings. To date, six symposia have been held by the ECH Sub committee on Drug Provings. As a result of this work, a Minimum Standard for Homoeopathic Drug Proving Protocols has been formulated as a consensus paper by delegates from nine European countries.

Section 2 has already been referred to in this text; the complete text of the Minimum Standards Protocols can be found in the Appendix.

One of the goals for the ECH Sub committee is:

- to integrate GHP and GHDP guidelines in the national drug laws (Good Homoeopathic Practice/Good Homoeopathic Drug Provings).

Tasks to be tackled during following meetings are:

- to coordinate activities among countries of Europe and also USA and South America
- to create consensus on Minimum Standards in conducting provings as well as on the education of proving doctors (European Committee for Homoeopathy, 1994), referring to the purpose of the proving.

Tasks in the area of documentation are:

- to create guidelines for documentation of designs and results in order to get comparable data
- to develop suitable software to integrate symptoms into materia medica
- to find criteria for confidence rating of symptoms, before they are integrated into the materia medica, e.g. number of times occurring in provings; number of cures; what does 'cured' mean in this context? etc.

Conclusion

A homoeopathic drug proving has to be understood as one of several pieces in a mosaic from which the complete drug picture is built. For the performance of a good homoeopathic drug proving the combination of a well-educated proving doctor, intimate supervision – essential during the first days of the proving – noting of the symptoms with meticulous precision and complete documentation of all events during the proving is necessary. The personal preference of the author is to aim for fewer high quality drug provings rather than a large quantity, because the practice of homoeopathic doctors shows that we do not use a large number of remedies so much as a core of well-understood remedies.

A 'happy relationship', a heart-to-heart contact between volunteer and proving doctor is the most essential prerequisite for good provings, even if this may not seem a very logical or scientific statement. But we should never forget that performing drug provings is an art as well as a science.

Appendix: Elements of a Minimum Standard For Homoeopathic Drug Proving Protocols (Version No. 2)

Introduction

A review of homoeopathic drug provings has shown that the methodology used for the different provings has been and still is extremely variable. Important items like the identity and source of the remedy and whether or not a placebo has been used, etc., often are not stated. In many cases it is not possible to find out which, if any, protocol has been followed during the proving. To meet today's standards of methodology, it is necessary to precisely describe the materials and methods of homoeopathic drug provings. The following eight point Minimum Standard has been developed by the Sub committee on Drug Provings as a consensus paper (delegates from nine countries have been involved in this process).

It should not be considered as a strict set of rules, but will help provide comparable results from provings which are conducted in Europe and elsewhere. The potencies and dosage given are not compulsory; the idea is to follow a given regimen for a period of time, e.g. 1–2 years, then compare the results and eventually change or amend the Standard according to the experiences of practice.

1. Qualification of the providing doctor:
   (a) minimum five years experience in homoeopathic practice,
   (b) to have personally proved a minimum of three remedies (as a volunteer).
2. Case taking (before pre-observation phase), case taking is obligatory:
   (a) for the safety of the volunteer, to make sure that they are healthy enough to take part in a proving,
   (b) to give a baseline of the actual state of health and symptoms,
   (c) to make sure that the volunteer has properly understood the purpose and procedure of the proving, is reliable (S126 Organon) and is able to express their symptoms precisely enough.
3. Inclusion criteria: The volunteers must be healthy in the sense that they do not show severe psychic or physical symptoms and do not consider themselves to be in need of medical treatment. The proving doctor should not see a necessity for treatment either.
4. Exclusion criteria: Pregnancy, breast feeding, allopathic treatments or homoeopathic drugs, contraceptive pills (intrauterine pessaries often contain cuprum, etc.; mark in the accounts).

5. Pre-observation period: not less than one week before intake of remedy, with recording of symptoms occurring during that time.
6. Drug administration:
   (a) Definition of the remedy: origin and identification, way of manufacturing (e.g. fresh plant, trituration or mother tincture, way of potentization, solvent, etc.).
   (b) Dosage and potency: normally C12 or C30, three globules every two hours (if another application form or dosage is given, please explain), as long as no symptoms occur, maximum six times, during one day, stop drug intake immediately if symptoms occur!
7. Documentation of symptoms:
   (a) Duration of observation of symptoms: minimum four weeks.
   (b) Supervision: intense contact between proving doctor and volunteer has to be secured, i.e. daily phonecalls, schedule of meetings.
   (c) Symptoms should include location, sensation, modality (time), concomitants and chronological records (illustrating how long after the commencement of the proving each symptom arose) and should be presented following the head to foot scheme, in distinct categories: 1) new, 2) old symptoms, 3) altered symptoms, 4) cured symptoms (Sherr, 1994).
   Complete original notes should be kept from each volunteer and proving doctor.
8. The legal requirements of a country must be considered.

References

Bayr, G. (1983) Eine Prüfung von Berberis vulgaris D3 und D30,1. Teil. AHZ., **228,** 177–86.

Dhawale, M.L. (1985) Principles and Practice of Homoeopathy. Bombay Institute of Clinical Research.

European Committee for Homoeopathy (1994) Homoeopathy in Europe. Sections 5–25. Paper can be ordered from Dr Jacques Imberechts, 134, Boulevard Leopold II B.1080 Brussels, Belgium.

Hahnemann, S. (reprint 1986) *Organon of Medicine*, 6th ed. Translated by W. Boericke. New Delhi-B. Jain Publishers.

Hering, C. (1974) *Guiding Symptoms of Our Materia Medica*, Vol. 1, Preface. New Delhi-B. Jain Publishers.

Hering, C. (1971) *Guiding Symptoms of Our Materia Medica*, Vol. 6. New Delhi-B. Jain Publishers.

Jansen, J.P. (1995) New Materia Medica. *Homoeopathic Links*, **1,** 33–4.

Kent, J.T. (reprint 1977) *Lectures on Homoeopathic Philosophy.* New Delhi-B. Jain Publishers.

Mezger, J. (1970) Eine neue Arzneimittelprüfung von Asarum Europaeum, (1.Teil). AHZ., **3,** 98–111.

Nagpaul, V.M. (1987) Provings – Planning and protocol. *British Homoeopathic Journal*, **76,** 76–80.

Riley, D. (1996) Homöopathische Arzneimittelprüfungen – Grundlagen und Praxis. Homint R&D Newsletter.

Sherr, J. (1994) *The Dynamics and Methodology of Homoeopathic Provings.* West Malvern, Dynamis Books.

Walach, H. (1992) Wissenschaftliche homöopathische Arzneimittelprüfung. Heidelberg, Haug.

Wieland, F. (1996) Is a Homoeopathic Drug Proving Just a Clinical Trial Phase One? *Homoeopathic Links*, **9,** 39–40.

Chapter 5

A systematic review of homoeopathic pathogenetic trials ('provings') published in the United Kingdom from 1945 to 1995*

Flávio Dantas and Peter Fisher

Introduction

Homoeopathy is a form of medicine, based on experiment, established by Hahnemann 200 years ago, mainly as a result of the testing of medicines in healthy volunteers and then applying the results to clinical practice on the basis of *Similia similibus curentur*–Let like cure like. This experimental testing, called *prüfung* in German – translated into nineteenth-century English as proving and recently, more accurately termed homoeopathic pathogenetic trial (Dantas, 1996)[1] – represents a unique and pioneering contribution of homoeopathy to medical knowledge.

The careful investigation of the pathogenetic properties of medicines was a fundamental principle in Hahnemann's work. He defined very precise guidelines for the conduct of HPTs. These included rules for selection of volunteers, preparation of medicine, minimization of confounding factors and criteria to select effects associated with the medicine. Hahnemann recognized the main methodological problems early, in his magnum opus, the *Organon* (1982). The issues he identified were: truthfulness of volunteers (§126), the use of medicines with differing potencies (§121) and individual differences (§129). To minimize these, he took several measures including the selection of trustworthy and conscientious human healthy volunteers (friends and sympathizers of homoeopathy), use of only one medicine in its purest form and in moderate doses, close supervision of the subjects and recommendations for controlling confounding variables such as diet, life style, ingestion of medicines and consumption of alcohol and caffeine-containing drinks.

Subsequently, many HPTs have been conducted using new designs and incorporating new methodologies using Hahnemann's original design – observation of effects with no comparative group – and applying his guidelines. In the last 50 years many improvements have been implemented in medical research in order to minimize the occurrence of bias and to

* This chapter is part of a systematic review of homoeopathic pathogenetic trials published from 1945 to 1995 in six languages – Dutch, English, French, German, Portuguese and Spanish – under the coordination of the first author. More than 150 reports were analysed and the results are to be published in a specialized journal.

improve the quality of inferences drawn from medical data. Among others, special mention should be given to the introduction of randomized controlled trials (RCTs) in medicine, dating back to 1948 with the streptomycin trial in Britain (Medical Research Council, 1948). Since then RCTs have become the standard design for drawing valid conclusions on efficacy of medicines (Altman, 1996).

The role of information gathered from HPTs and the methodology of HPTs have been recently discussed by the homoeopathic community. In the EU the Subcommittee on Drug Proving of the European Committee for Homoeopathy is formulating minimum standards for homoeopathic pathogenetic trial protocols. In USA the Council on Pharmacy of the Homeopathic Pharmacopoeia Convention of the United States sponsored a workshop on the methodology of HPTs in 1995. In the United Kingdom, Brazil and India, countries where homoeopathy is part of the public health system, HPTs are being conducted by official institutions or academic departments in public hospitals. The role of information gathered from HPTs is also relevant to clarify the process of registration and regulation of homoeopathic medicines by official regulatory bodies.

Overviews of the medical literature according to predefined criteria has been one of the tools used in medicine to synthesize data into meaningful and unified sets. It is a young and controversial area in the medical literature, which has been in continuous development in the last 10 years. The poor scientific quality of reviews of clinical research was exposed in 1987 in a seminal paper by Mulrow (1987). Several terminological discussions have taken place at academic meetings and in the specialized literature of clinical epidemiology on the subject of meta-analysis and systematic reviews. Among other proposals, Anello and Fleiss (1995) suggested a distinction between studies which aim to estimate a common effect size and studies intended to pose and answer new questions. They called the former type of study analytic meta-analysis and the latter, focusing on the characteristics of the studies which account for the observed differences in the reported effect sizes, exploratory meta-analysis.

Our systematic review focuses on the characteristics of the different HPTs published in the UK in the last 50 years. As this is a qualitative overview we are particularly concerned with critical examination of the effects reported from HPTs, including an analysis of their methodological rigour and reliability, and in informally exploring the possible sources of variability among study results.

To what extent have HPTs incorporated new methods developed in experimental medicine in the last 50 years? Can we rely on the conclusions drawn from HPTs done during this period? Have they being conducted according to the ethical standards established since the Nuremburg Code of 1947? How informative and reproducible are the publications on HPTs in the literature? To our knowledge there is no systematic summary of data or search for patterns in HPTs which addresses these questions. We therefore conducted a systematic review of reports of HPTs published in the United Kingdom from 1945 to 1995 in order to assess the methodological quality of HPTs and to help investigators in designing future HPTs.

HPTs: basic definitions and historical overview

In essence an HPT is a clinical trial to investigate the effects of potentially toxic or pathogenic substances, diluted and attenuated according to homoeopathic pharmacopoeias, in non-patient volunteers in good and relatively stable health conditions. Historically, HPTs are the first systematic, experimental approach to detecting changes in healthy volunteers after exposure to a drug. They are similar in conception to Phase 1 clinical trials according to the FDA regulations developed in the 1960s but were developed over 150 years earlier.

A homoeopathic medicine is a substance which is potentially toxic or pathogenic, prepared according to the specifications of an homoeopathic pharmacopoeia (including trituration or dilution and succussion). An HPT aims to produce *valid* and *useful* data concerning objective and subjective changes at mental, general or local levels, provoked by an homoeopathic medicine in apparently healthy human beings.

The information gathered from HPTs, together with data from toxicological sources and clinical experience after using the medicine, is used to build a data-set to be compared with the symptoms an individual patient is experiencing. From this comparison follows a decision on the medicine most likely to provoke similar symptoms in human beings, thus applying the basic assumption of homoeopathy – let like cure like.

The critical importance of HPTs can be deduced from the need for a correct comparison between the concrete symptoms the patient presents with the supposedly reliable symptoms reported in homoeopathic materia medica, many of them originating in HPTs. Hahnemann was very concerned with this aspect and the ethical consequences of misconduct in this area. He even wrote that 'anybody publishing the results of such experiments for the medical world becomes responsible for the reliability of the experimental subject and the accuracy of his reports, and rightly so, since the well-being of suffering mankind is at stake' (Note to §139). He also advised against paying healthy volunteers to participate in homoeopathic trials and tried to dissuade doctors from doing long distance or mail trials on the grounds of unreliability and uncertainty of results (§143).

In the first edition of the *Organon of the Rational Art of Healing* (1810), Hahnemann asserted that 'the rational nature of the art of medicine manifests itself pre-eminently in the rejection of all systematic and other prejudices, in the refusal to act without good grounds, in the adoption of every possible measure to achieve the desired action, and in confining attention as much as possible to that which can be definitely ascertained' (1913; §47).

For Hahnemann, a true materia medica should be a collection of the authentic, pure, reliable effects of simple medicinal substances in themselves (§143) where all conjecture, everything merely asserted or entirely fabricated, should be completely excluded (1982; §144). He also stated that 'the curative virtues of medicines cannot be apprehended by specious a priori sophistry, or from the smell, taste, or appearance of the medicines, or from chemical analysis, or by treating disease with one or more of them in a mixture' (1982; §110).

Prevention of guess-work, imagination and recording of findings only after close questioning were continuously stressed in different editions of the *Organon*. Only reliable symptoms should be included in the homoeopathic materia medica: that is the clear message present in all the editions of Hahnemann's *Organon*. Hahnemann would not permit transgression of this golden rule in the search for knowledge of the 'individual disease-producing powers of medicines which are to act as counter-diseases for the cure of natural diseases' (1913; §38). He was, 200 years ago, in tune with the current movement for evidence-based medicine and better medical research.

In attempting to minimize the effects of suggestion on volunteers Hahnemann recommended that 'in the investigation of these drug-symptoms all suggestion must be as rigidly avoided as in the examination of the symptoms of disease' (1913; §115). To obtain symptoms as accurately as possible, every subject had a pocket-size notebook to write down the sensations and changes immediately after they occurred. The volunteers were required to repeat the description of the changes without referring to this notebook during the personal interview: if the accounts varied he advised the director of the trial to confront the subject with both versions and invite him to choose and confirm the statement which is nearest to the truth (1982; §116).

Hahnemann met the subjects participating in his trials, mostly friends and attendees at his lectures (Haehl, 1983), every day or every two or three days to interrogate them about their symptoms. He was aware of the impossibility of absolutely and perfectly healthy volunteers and also recommended writing in brackets slight ailments to allow volunteers to indicate that they were dubious or not confirmed (Hahnemann, 1936). He also recommended, in the Preface to his *Materia Medica Pura,* rejection of all symptoms developed after some extraordinary circumstance which might be supposed to alter the results.

Methods

Search strategy for identifying relevant studies

The search of published trials was performed by manual searching of books and journals, scanning reference lists and expert knowledge complemented by information from bibliographic databases (HOMINFORM – British Library of Homoeopathy). The *British Homoeopathic Journal* was hand-searched from 1945 to 1995 by one of us (FD).

Selection criteria

Inclusion

Only published reports of HPTs were included, irrespective of the number of volunteers, experimental design or outcome measures used to assess the effects of the medicine. We included reports of trials using diluted and potentized homoeopathic medicines with the aim of detecting changes in healthy volunteers[2] as a result of the exposure to a specific homoeopathic medicine. Publications of all kinds were included: books, proceedings of congresses and homoeopathic meetings held in the UK (regional, national and international) and journals published in the UK from 1945 to 1995. The decision on inclusion was made by the authors after referring to the review protocol. Only written information in the public domain was accepted.

Exclusion
Publications dealing only with theoretical or methodological aspects of HPTs and not reporting any experimental results were excluded. Translated reports of HPTs were also excluded; they will be included in an international systematic review, analysed in the language of their original publication. Multiple publications of the same data were also checked and excluded. Reports of trials dealing exclusively with mother tinctures were excluded.[3]

Methods of assessment

Each report was analysed independently by the two authors according to predefined criteria using a standard form comprising 86 questions and a final open question for methodological criticisms. The form was designed to collect relevant information on the setting, population, design, outcomes, assessment and interpretation of results of HPT reports. For every report we collected bibliographic details, description of the setting, substance tested, method of preparation, volunteers included in the study, details of the study design, assessment of outcomes, presentation and interpretation of results and personal synthetic appraisal. Withdrawal rates, study methodology, presence of adverse effects, percentage of sensitive volunteers and number of claims from each HPT were also extracted. The information quality of the reports was assessed using a separate form completed by one of us (FD).

Development of the data-extraction form

A draft of the assessment form was developed by the first author with further comments and suggestions by the second author. It comprised 75 items and was sent to reviewers who agreed to participate in our international study for further comments and suggestions. A second form with 79 items was then designed and sent to all reviewers for a pilot study using three reports of HPTs originally published in English. These three reports were selected on the basis of their methodological differences: one was a self-experiment, another a randomized double-blind placebo controlled trial using different dilutions of the same medicine and the third a randomized double-blind placebo controlled trial of one medicine in a specific dilution. Again suggestions and comments were incorporated in the final version of the form.

The data-extraction form was designed to give, first, an analytical perspective of the studies regarding their validity and, second, a more elaborate objective and subjective overall judgement on methodological quality and clinical utility based on absolute and relative opinions.

Content of the form

For each medicine the name, dilution(s), method of dilution, presentation, dose, frequency per day, repetition of doses, total duration of the trial, number of active treatment periods and duration per volunteer (in days), source of the drug, mode of preparation and preparation responsibility was recorded. Regarding the study population we extracted the initial and final number, ethnic origin, sex, age, occupation, number of control volunteers, percentage of sensitive volunteers, inclusion criteria, exclusion criteria, assessment of health status prior to admission, training of volunteers, personality traits, physical characteristics, informed consent and method of recruitment.

The study method was assessed in terms of: approval of protocol by Ethical Committee, direction/coordination, randomization, sequence generation of subjects in the trial, allocation concealment, masking (blindness) of volunteers and of supervisor, use of placebo, pre-trial observation period with or without placebo, placebo distinguishable from verum, placebo potentized, comparative group, crossover, washout period (post-treatment observation), management of adverse effects, rules for stopping medicine. The assessment of each trial was recorded in terms of: use of symptom diary, type of diary, initial interview (case-taking/collection of previous symptoms), follow-up interview, use of laboratory investigations, use of psychological tests, withdrawal/dropout of volunteers (losses to follow-up), reason for withdrawal, withdrawal due to severe adverse effects, presence of adverse effects and predefined categories for assessment of the attributes of a symptom.

For the presentation of results we extracted information on the frequency of symptoms in the sample, description of complete symptoms, analytical presentation, chronology of symptoms, character of symptoms, location of symptoms, duration of symptoms, onset of symptoms, intensity of symptoms, modalities of symptoms, presence of concomitant symptoms, inclusion of prior symptoms that improved during the trial, detailed report of individual volunteers, use of symptom tables and charts.

The interpretation of the results by the authors was reviewed in terms of: predefined criteria to include medicine effects, use of descriptive statistics (measures of central tendency or dispersion of data), use of statistical tests and presence and number of significant findings claimed.

Finally, each reviewer was invited to make a subjective judgement: 'after reading and analysing all the points above, and based exclusively on the published report':

- Do you think the symptoms stated as belonging to the medicine can be trusted?
- Would you apply the information given in it into your clinical practice to prescribe this medicine to a patient? For both questions the options were certainly, almost certainly, probably, possibly, with serious reservations, definitely not, can't answer or none claimed.
- From a methodological point of view, do you judge this report of proving as: completely reliable, very reliable, reliable, unreliable, completely unreliable?
- Compared to the other reports you have read, do you think this is: below average, average, above average, much above average, excellent?

A final open question asked about the main methodological criticisms of the reviewer to each study. During the final process of consensus reaching, all reviewers were asked to answer two additional questions regarding the rationale and source category of the substance tested in each trial.

Process of examination and resolution of disagreements

Data extraction was done independently by the two authors using our standard data-extraction sheet. Both reviewers are clinicians with experience in conducting randomized clinical trials or HPTs. The results were then entered on a database and the discrepancies were noted and discussed in order to reach a consensual answer. The number of findings or pathogenetic effects was counted. Some answers had to be partially estimated, for instance, adequate masking, distinguishability of placebo, incidence of symptoms in the sample and in a few reports the final number of included volunteers. The reviewers estimated these whenever adequate information was available in the report. The data were then revised and used for the synthetic picture of reported HPTs.

Grading of studies

The heterogeneity of methods and outcomes led us to develop summated and hierarchical indexes to grade studies in terms of methodological quality and degree of experimental control. The subjective methodological appraisal (SMA) index was based on the sum of the answers of the two reviewers to the questions on judgement from a methodological point of view and relative quality of the report compared to others. We awarded 4 points to trials judged 'completely reliable' and no points to trials appraised as 'completely unreliable'. The SMA index thus had 16 as maximum and 0 as minimum. The results were organized in four categories sorted by decreasing perception of quality (I best, II, III, IV in order of decreasing overall quality as judged by two reviewers). Category I included trials scoring 13 to 16; Category II, 9 to 12; Category III, 5 to 8 and Category IV, 0 to 4.

The experimental control (EC) index was developed as an hierarchical arrangement following currently accepted methodological criteria for assessing the quality of clinical trials. For instance papers including the description of randomization scored higher than non-randomized (or randomization 'not stated') HPTs. Other components of the index were: masking of supervisor and volunteers, use of comparative group and pre-observation period with or without placebo. Again the results were expressed in four categories with Class I being the most sound from a methodological perspective. The index is described in Table 5.1.

The agreement between the two reviewers was calculated using Kappa statistics. Based on the two indices we selected the best studies (studies included in Class I or II on both indices).

Magnitude of effects

We defined pathogenetic effects as all clinical events and laboratory findings noted by volunteers during an HPT and recorded in the final report. In other words they are the findings claimed at the end of the trial by authors

Table 5.1 Experimental Control index

	Volunteer masking	*Supervisor masking*	*Pre-observation period*	*Comparative group*	*Class*
Well described	yes	yes	yes	yes	I
Partially described or crossover studies	yes	yes/no	yes/no	yes	II (only one 'no')
Only stated	yes	no	no	yes	III
Not stated	yes/no	yes/no	yes/no	yes/no	IV

to be used by practitioners seeing patients with similar pictures. The overall incidence of pathogenetic effects in each trial was calculated by dividing the number of volunteers with at least one pathogenetic effect by the total number of volunteers taking the medicine and who definitely contributed to the final picture of the remedy. The incidence of pathogenetic effects per volunteer was defined as the total number of findings claimed in the trial divided by the total number of subjects using the medicine and included in its final pathogenetic description. It would have been more correct to use the total number of volunteers reporting at least one pathogenetic effect in the denominator but this information was partially or totally missing in 38% of the reports in our sample.

Therefore we decided to offer a range of values for these categories in which the first value is very conservative and without any estimation of the effect while the second is based on educated guess. For instance in one of the trials (12) the conservative value for the overall incidence of pathogenetic effects is 20%. This value reflects the lack of information on which volunteers reported each symptom: the paper only describes the total number of volunteers experiencing a particular symptom (and this was 4 in a sample of 20 taking verum). On the other hand 385 pathogenetic effects are reported and shared by this sample. Given the tradition in the area it is likely that all the volunteers experienced at least one symptom (100%), however, this cannot be categorically stated. We think giving minimum and maximum figures for trials in which relevant data for these categories were missing is the most informative option.

We counted as one pathogenetic effect a piece of information which could be included in an homoeopathic repertory as an independent subheading. For instance 'boring headache ameliorated by pressure' was counted as one claim. The use of this fractional symptom approach may explain – in some cases – the high number of claimed findings. When there was a summary of symptoms it was used to count the findings. In rare cases (31) there is an explicit statement by the author that all symptoms – even with slight variations – are reported, even at the risk of seeming repetitive.

Information quality of reports

One of us (FD) developed a form for evaluating the information quality of the reports. The form consists of ten questions concerning the most important information which should be present in a report. These are:

- rationale,
- criteria for inclusion and exclusion,
- information on the experimental/social setting,
- medicine tested,
- study design,
- assessment of outcomes,
- selection of pathogenetic effects,
- description of pathogenetic effects,
- summary of the magnitude of effects, and
- linking of results with other relevant studies.

The questions were framed as an ideal statement to which the respondent could agree or disagree after reading the particular topic in each report. For each question a scale with items in Likert response format was developed with three options for agree or disagree: slightly, moderately or strongly, plus a not applicable alternative, giving a total of seven options. We attributed '0' to not applicable and '1' to slightly disagree going up to '6' (strongly agree). The score thus ranged from 10 to 60. Three reports were randomly selected from each of the five decades from 1945 to 1995 and analysed by one of the authors (FD). In total 15 reports were analysed.

Statistical procedures

We made extensive use of descriptive statistics, charts and visual data plots – to inform as much raw data as possible – instead of inferential statistics due to the exploratory character of the review. Kappa statistics was used to evaluate agreement between reviewers judging methodological quality of the trials and concordance between methodological indexes.

Results

Forty-five reports of trials reporting the effects of 44 different medicines in 779 volunteers were analysed. The trials were published mainly in homoeopathic journals (84%, all but one in the *British Homoeopathic Journal*), 11% in books and 5% in conference proceedings. Twenty-two different investigators contributed as first author, with two individuals accounting for 42% of the total. In total 7043 pathogenetic effects or findings were claimed for the medicines studied. Twenty-five HPTs were done with medicines never previously tested. The medicines were tested in 24 different dilutions – mostly centesimal (71%) and decimal (29%). The most frequently used dilution in our sample was 30c (24%) followed by 6c (17%) and 12c (14%). In 28 trials more than one dilution was used, 17 of the trials used one dilution only. Active homoeopathic medicines were tested in 641 volunteers and placebo in 177 volunteers.[4] The number of HPTs per decade is shown in Table 5.2.

Table 5.3 shows the characteristics of studies included in our review.

Table 5.2 Number of HPTs per decade included in the review (1945 to 1995)

Year	*Number of published HPTs*
1945–1955	8
1956–1965	10
1966–1975	11
1976–1985	7
1986–1995	9

Information quality

Much vital information for the analysis and reproducibility of HPTs was missing in a substantial number of reports. For instance the medicine, its preparation and dosage was often not adequately described. The source of the substance used in the trials was completely described and fully reproducible in only 7% of reports and partially described in 56%. In 36% of the reports the source was not stated and in one trial it was unknown (Carcinosinum). The mode of preparation of the medicine was not described in 73% of the reports. We were especially interested in information useful for designing future HPTs, in particular the pattern of pathogenetic effects such as time of appearance after exposure to the medicine, severity and duration of the symptoms – but this information was lacking in three-quarters of the trials.

In the overall evaluation of the quality of the reports the mean score was 35.5 (SD 8.9). The weakest features were the grounds on which pathogenetic effects were selected and associated with the medicine (mean 1.7, SD 1.1). The rationale for testing the substance achieved the maximum rank among the ten items, it was well described in most of the publications. This finding is consistent with the information found to be missing in individual analysis of the reports.

The reporting of pathogenetic effects in books was more extensive (mean 632 effects) than in journals (98) or conference proceedings (71). The effects were usually presented following the schema of Kent's Repertory or arranged by anatomical regions.

Rationale

The most frequent reason for selection of substances for an HPT was known medicinal properties, followed by known toxic effects in humans. In 13% of the reports the rationale for selection of the substance was not described. Figure 5.1 shows the distribution of different rationales used to test substances in our sample.

In a few trials the authors tried to identify an association between the pathogenetic effects using high dilutions and substantial doses but in general this was not done. Some non-toxic substances were tested often on the basis of a symbolic relationship, e.g. the edible bird-nest used in Chinese cookery as a possible remedy for child abuse (5).

Table 5.3 Features of studies included in review of HPTs published in the UK (1945–1995)

Trial	*Tested medicine*	*Country*	*Study design (duration in weeks)*	*Sample size*	*Incidence*	
					Overall (estimated)	*Per volunteer*
	Plant					
Chand 1982[2]	Cassia sophera MT, 30c, 200c	IND	Uncontrolled (?)	?	?	?
Clover 1980[3]	Pulsatilla 3x	UK	Crossover (12)	18	0	0
Julian 1964[7]	Nepenthes 3x, 6x, 15x	FRA	Parallel (?)	?	?	?
McIvor 1980[10]	Phormium tenax 6c, 30c	NZL	Uncontrolled (21)	1	100	63
McIvor 1975[11]	Gingko biloba 6c	NZL	Uncontrolled (10)	1	100	24
O'Hanlon 1952[13]	Strophantus sarmentosus 6c, 12c, 30c	UK	Uncontrolled	8	100	6.9
Pratt 1971[16]	Lycopodium, Rhus tox, Spigelia 200 and Mag-p 200 (mineral)	UK	Parallel (6)	103	20 (a)	0.2
Raeside 1960[18]	Triosteum perfoliatum 8c	UK	Parallel (?)	15	54	16
Raeside 1965[22]	Luffa operculata 6c, 12c, 30c	UK	Parallel (2)	13	15 (77)	9.7
Raeside 1966[23]	Mandragora officinarum 3x, 6x, 12x	UK	Uncontrolled (2)	18	83 (100)	6
Raeside 1967[24]	Colchicum autumnale 6x, 6c, 30c	UK	Uncontrolled (2)	17	88 (100)	5.8
Raeside 1969[26]	Lophophitum leandri 6x, 6c, 12c	UK	Uncontrolled (2)	11	91 (100)	5.8
Raeside 1971[27]	Mimosa pudica 6x, 6c, 9c, 12c, 30c	UK	Uncontrolled (2)	21	95 (100)	4.6
Riley 1995[28]	Veronica officinalis 12c	USA	Parallel (8)	17	100	7.7
Sankaran 1970[30]	Mimosa pudica 3x, 6x	IND	Parallel (4)	6	50	4.8
Sherr 1993[32]	Chocolate 6c, 12c, 30c, 100c, 200c	UK	Parallel (?)	15	100	60
Templeton 1952[38]	Strophantus sarmentosus 2x, 3x, 6c, 12c, 30c	UK	Crossover (6)	7	100	11
Templeton 1956[42]	Rauwolfia serpentina 3x, 6x, 12c, 30c	UK	Parallel (26)	10	?	18
Vakil 1989[43]	Iris versicolor 3c	IND	Parallel (3)	16	80	2.6
Walach 1993[45]	Belladonna 30c	GER	Crossover (10)	45	29	0
	Animal					
Engel 1975[5]	Nidus edulis 3x, 4x, 6x, 10x, 12x, 15x, 20x, 30x	UK	Parallel (2)	23	100	1.7
Houghton 1995[6]	Lac humanum 30c	UK	Parallel (?)	13	85	27
Nagpaul 1989[12]	Tarantula hispanica 6c, 30c, 200c	IND	Parallel (12)	28	20 (~100)	19
Raeside 1959[17]	Hydrophis cyanocinctus 6c, 30c	UK	Parallel (12)	14	100	8.5
Raeside 1962[20]	Venus mercenaria 6c, 12c, 30c	UK	Parallel (2)	19	68 (100)	7
Raeside 1964[21]	Hirudo medicinalis 6x, 6c, 30c	UK	Parallel (2)	18	67	7.3

Table 5.3 *continued*

Trial	*Tested medicine*	*Country*	*Study design (duration in weeks)*	*Sample size*	*Incidence*	
					Overall (estimated)	*Per volunteer*
Sankaran 1970[29]	Atrax robustus 30c	IND	Parallel (9)	4	33	8.7
Sherr 1985[31]	Androctonus ammorrexi 50C	UK	Parallel (?)	31	100	24
	Mineral/chemical element					
Julian 1983[8]	Plantinum 4c, 7c, 30c	FRA	Parallel (?)	60	?	7.1
Raeside 1961[19]	Selenium 6c, 12c, 30c	UK	Parallel (4)	21	38 (?100)	7.7
Raeside 1968[25]	Tellurium 6x, 6c, 12c	UK	Uncontrolled (2)	17	76 (100)	5.1
Sherr 1992[33]	Hydrogen 6c, 9c, 12c, 15c, 30c, 200c	UK	Parallel (?)	18	100	73
Smith 1979[34]	Kali carbonicum 6c, 30c, 200c	UK	Parallel (8)	9	100	21
Templeton 1949[35]	Cadmium metallicum 2c	UK	Uncontrolled (?)	9	100	17
Templeton 1953[39]	Beryllium metallicum 3x, 6x, 7x, 12x, 30x	UK	Parallel (?)	11	?(?100)	17
Vakil 1988[44]	Iodum 12x	IND	Uncontrolled (3)	8	?	(b)
	Chemicals					
Templeton 1949[36]	Alloxan 2c, 6c, 30c	UK	Parallel (9)	17	100	7.7
Templeton 1951[37]	Alloxan 1x, 3x, 12c	UK	Parallel (17)	16	100	24
	Medicinal drugs/use					
Kenyon 1947[9]	Penicillin calcium 12c	UK	Parallel (7)	5	20	2.4
Pai 1965[14]	Chlorpromazine 30c	IND	Parallel (?)	16	92	2.0
Pai 1967[15]	Tetanus toxin 30c	IND	Parallel (6)	14	91	5.2
Templeton 1956[41]	Cortisone and ACTH 30x, 6c, 12c, 30c	UK	Parallel (?)	22	?(?100)	11
	Energy					
Chakravarty 1982[1]	Solar eclipse ray 3x	IND	Parallel (3)	15	87	3.4
Daws 1992[4]	Sol britannic 30c	UK	Parallel (?)	12	92	26
	Nosode					
Templeton 1954[40]	Carcinosin 30c, 200c	UK	Parallel (?)	17	?	7.3

(a) No pathogenetic effect was reported for 28 volunteers taking Magnesia phosphorica 200
(b) Can't calculate (laboratory findings collectively analysed)

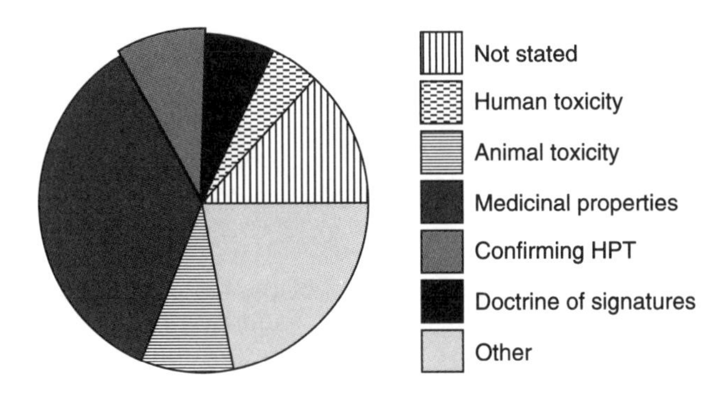

Figure 5.1 Rationale for conducting reported HPTs.

Settings

Most HPTs were done in homoeopathic teaching or research centres under the supervision of medical doctors. The information in the reports generally does not give a clear picture of the setting but the trials conducted in London between 1947 and 1971 were done with students of homoeopathy. HPTs were mostly done in the context of homoeopathic courses with friendly, and subordinate, volunteers. The possibility of intercommunication between volunteers and possible contamination of results by suggestion was raised and measures taken to prevent this were described in some reports (3, 5, 19).

Supervision

Most investigators were homoeopathic physicians but in the last 10 years non-medically qualified practitioners (NMQPs), NMQP students and other health professionals (such as clinical psychologists) have supervised some HPTs. Only 27% of the reports described an initial interview with volunteers (illness history, current complaints or medical interview) rarely specifying its duration or specific contents. The use of follow-up interviews was not stated on 76% of the reports. Three of the four best trials were done without direct contact between the supervisor and volunteers during the trial (only in the first instance was there personal contact between the supervisor and potential volunteers). These HPTs generally yielded very few or no statistically significant pathogenetic effects. In the other one volunteers were interrogated daily as far as possible, reporting an average of 19.3 pathogenetic findings per volunteer, but no statistical analysis was applied comparing placebo and verum effects.

Ethical aspects

Many HPTs did not conform to modern ethical standards. Informed consent was not mentioned in 91%, Ethical Committee approval was explicitly referred to in only one report. Students from other countries attending homoeopathic courses were the preferred sample in London in the 1960s. Payment of volunteers was indirectly reported, in the acknowledgement of a funding body, in five publications (23–27).

Population

Inclusion criteria were not stated in 76% of the reports. When stated they were based mostly on clinical history (29%) and laboratory findings (20%). The assessment of health status prior to admission of volunteers was not reported in 67% of the trials. Poor inclusion criteria for volunteers was tacitly acknowledged in the report of the HPT of Hirudo medicinalis where one volunteer had an haemoptysis and was admitted to hospital, bronchiectasis was eventually diagnosed (21). Most of the volunteers were students of homoeopathy or people with some knowledge of homoeopathy. In general there is a description of the gender and age of the volunteers but information on ethnicity is lacking.

Study design

Most of the studies used parallel group (64%) or uncontrolled designs (29%), some more recent studies have used crossover designs (7%). Randomization was described in 13% of the reports (the first randomized HPT was reported in 1961 (19)). Masking of volunteers only (single-blind) was applied in 13% of the HPTs, 24% were double-blind. Pre-observation period without placebo was reported in two trials, seven had a placebo run-in phase.

Comparative group and placebo control

Placebo was used in 29 trials. A placebo run-in phase was reported in 16% of the trials. Placebo was definitely indistinguishable from active medicine in 9% of reports; in 22% it was distinguishable. In total, 27% of the volunteers took placebo. Placebo was used for various purposes: as comparative controls, as a device to increase the awareness of volunteers and in an intermediate way whereby symptoms generated by volunteers taking placebo were used for elimination. Placebo was used and its symptoms were described by the two most prolific authors of reports in their first trials but on later reports they do not describe the placebo symptoms and in one case, even abandoned its use as unhelpful. The leading author in the 1960s stated, in his first report (17), that 'the symptoms produced by this drug were, on the whole, clear and impressive, with a conformity which was completely absent in the controls. Strangely enough some of the controls had night starts and even sore throats, but a glance through the books shows at once which is "prover" and which control'.

We searched for references or patterns of placebo and pathogenetic effects in our sample. Some of them state that nothing at all happened with placebo or that events did not follow a significant pattern, and that this was a confirmation that any symptoms which were noted could be attributed to the tested medicine. Others argued that 'controls were an unnecessary waste of good provers' and that 'in our particular type of work they are rather pointless, as we believe that it has been shown beyond reasonable doubt that the symptoms used in making the final proving picture do not occur significantly in control students' (22). The better-controlled trials used placebo as a comparative group for statistical analysis. In general, they compare event days or number of changes per day in volunteers using placebo and verum. The possibility that placebo controls did produce symptoms similar to volunteers using verum – and how to assess them – was posed in the discussion of one of the reports (19), the author acknowledged it would be possible to make a 'drug picture' from the control symptoms but argued that placebo symptoms 'were never severe, nor were they constant in one control, nor in the various controls when their symptoms were compared'. Although placebo was reportedly used in 26 trials where no statistical analysis was applied only three of them presented a description of the symptoms produced by placebo volunteers.

Duration

The median duration of the trials was 34 days. It was difficult in some cases to estimate the precise duration of the trial as important details were missing. In some cases there was a long follow-up of some volunteers, as long as ten months (6).

Sample size

Mean sample size was 17.8, range 1–103 (SD 16.5). Three studies were done with one volunteer, the author of the report. Some trials using different dilutions used the same volunteers (in this review we have counted each volunteer only once). Low methodological quality studies used smaller sample sizes than better studies, as shown in Figure 5.2.

The evolution of methodological quality of the trials published from 1945 to 1995 shows some improvement, but a much greater diversity of quality in more recent studies. Figure 5.3 illustrates this evolution.

Methodological quality

Most HPTs were of low methodological quality (see Figure 5.4 in terms of experimental control or subjective methodological appraisal index). The level of agreement between the two reviewers for the SMA index was moderate (Kappa = 0.51, 95% CI 0.38–0.64). The concordance between the results of EC and SMA indexes was also moderate (Kappa = 0.48, 95% CI 0.34–0.62).

Trials of poor methodological quality (Classes III or IV) yielded more pathogenetic effects than trials of better quality (Classes I or II). Figure 5.5 shows the mean number of pathogenetic effects per volunteers by class.

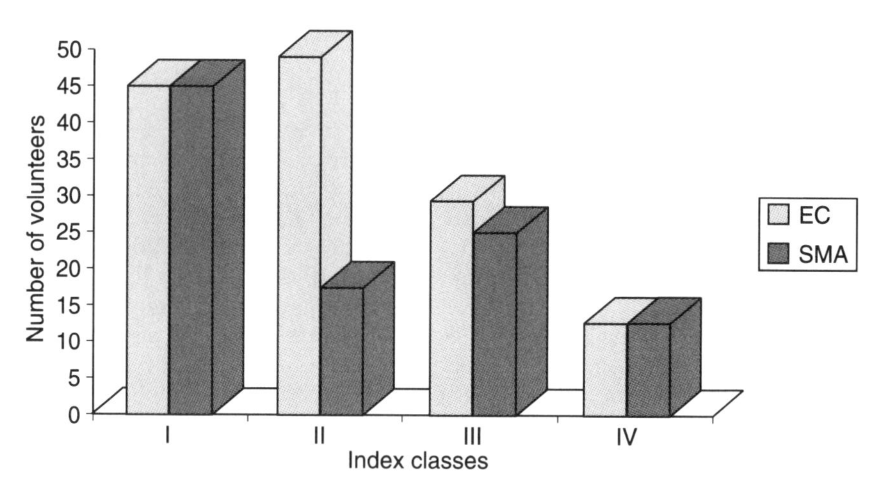

Figure 5.2 Mean number of volunteers by index classes.

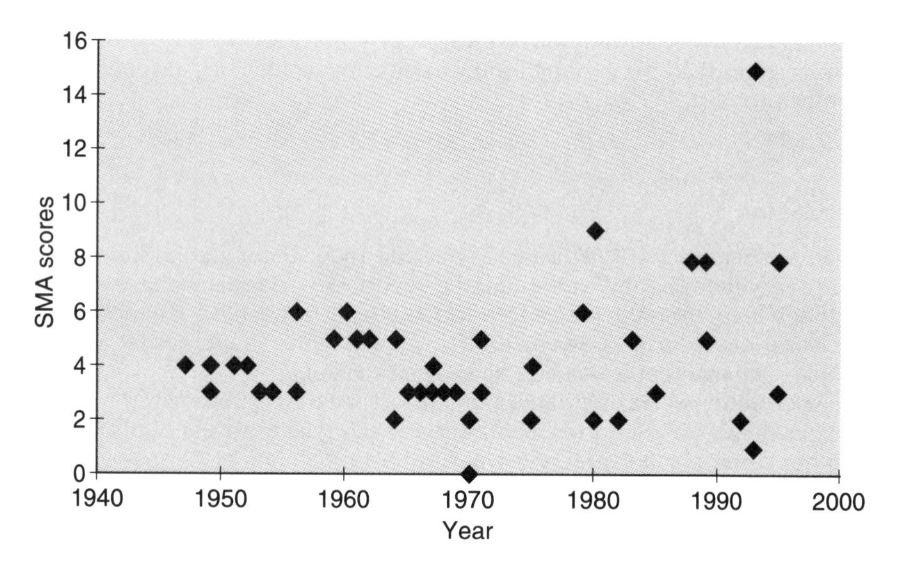

Figure 5.3 SMA scores across time.

Clinical usefulness

Both reviewers judged the clinical applicability of reported HPTs as not outstanding. Considering the overall judgement one of the reviewers would 'possibly' apply the information given in the reports and the other would

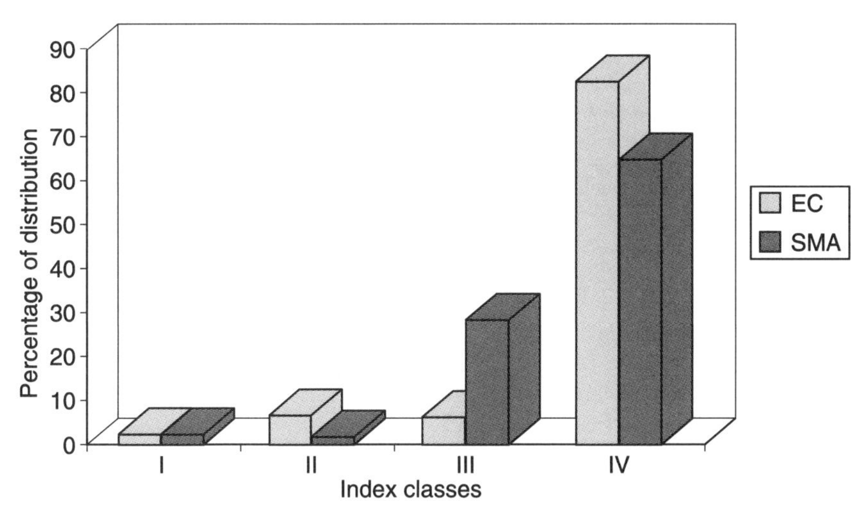

Figure 5.4 Distribution (in %) of reports by index classes.

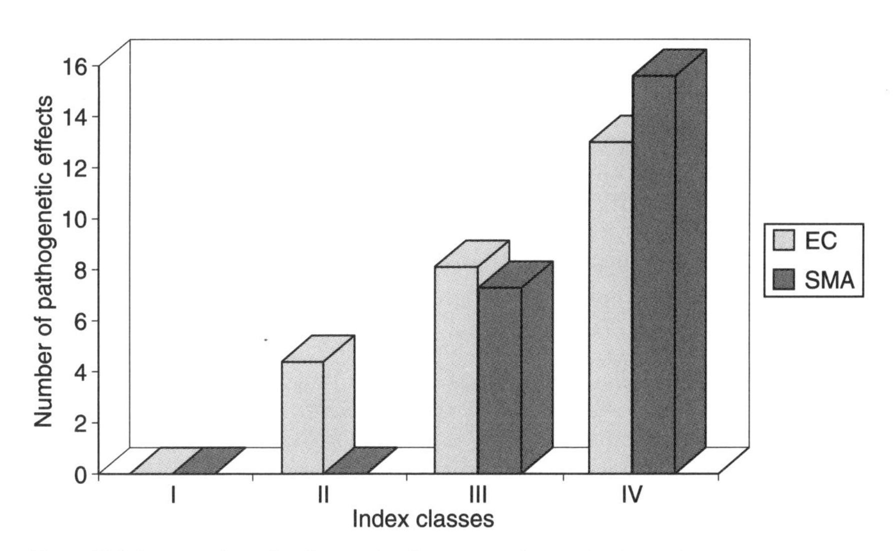

Figure 5.5 Mean number of pathogenetic effects per volunteer by index classes.

apply 'with serious reservations'. Although in only six reports there was a disagreement between more than one category, the final agreement between reviewers for this question was fair (Kappa = 0.30, 95% CI 0.16–0.44).

Table 5.4 Characteristics of trials by authors with three or more published reports

Author	*Year*	*Number of reports*	*Symptom selection criteria*	*Healthy volunteer criteria*	*Use of placebo*	*Mean incidence per volunteer*
A	1949–1956	8	no	in 50%	initially	14.0
B	1959–1971	11	no	no	initially	7.5
C	1985–1993	3	no	no	yes – not for comparison	52.5

Effects

Incidence

All but one HPT reported pathogenetic effects or some difference between placebo and verum irrespective of the medicine or dilution used.[5] The mean overall incidence of pathogenetic effects – excluding trials with less than five volunteers using verum – was 76.7% in our conservative calculation or 85.1% after estimation. The mean incidence of pathogenetic effects per volunteer was 19.2 (7043/366) using a conservative method or 18.2 (7043/386) by a more probable estimate. The incidence of pathogenetic effects was clearly associated with the methodological quality of studies: better studies generally claimed few or no significant effects, poor studies claimed a large number of effects. Overall there was an average of 156 effects per trial (SD 212.0), range 0–1100.

It is notable that, when attempts to use statistical methods to compare the incidence of symptoms in verum and placebo, the results were uncertain or negative. On the other hand, where the only criterion was supervisor judgement, all studies yielded some pathogenetic effects. Table 5.4 illustrates findings collected from authors publishing three or more reports in our sample.

Pathogenethic effects

Nature

There was a huge diversity in the nature of reported effects. Mental, general, cravings and aversions, dreams and local symptoms were described. In general the reports did not summarize the number of symptoms by area but there were notable similarities and contrasts between the patterns described. For instance, the author of an HPT of *Luffa operculata* commented on the great similarity of results of trials in Britain and in Germany. But for *Lophophytum leandri* there was a complete absence of mental symptoms in the German trial while the British one had quite marked mental symptoms.

A superficial view indicates the high incidence of common and general symptoms such as irritability, depression, headaches, skin changes, sleep and gastrointestinal symptoms. For instance, *Kali carbonicum* produced six marked symptoms: lassitude, weakness, fatigue, lack of energy, feeling tired and sleepy during the day and depression. One wonders after reading the reports if cultural factors do not play an important role in the choice of symptoms by volunteers and subsequent reporting (e.g. the British preoccupation with bowel function).

Latency

In nine trials there was information on the time of occurrence of symptoms after exposure to the medicine. Most events occurred in the first week after taking the medicine but there are isolated reports of symptoms appearing many weeks after starting the trial (33).

Duration

Very little information was recorded. Only one paper presented complete information on the duration of all pathogenetic effects and placebo symptoms (36). In this report most of the symptoms have a short duration (up to 7 days) and the longest lasted for 31 days.

Severity

Again, very little information is available. There was a varying degree of symptom severity but the information was not systematically collected or clearly presented in the reports.

Dilution-response relationship

There is no basis for extracting valid information on this point. One of the most experienced investigators conducted trials using different dilutions of the same substances in separate terms. He concluded that in general, but not always, better results were obtained in the final term irrespective of the dilution used. We could not find evidence that high dilutions yield more mental symptoms than low ones.

Given the widely varying characteristics of the trials, it is methodologically unsound to search for consistency of effects in different reports of the same substance being tested in several dilutions. Even the comparison among the top four trials cannot help us in addressing this important question because the substances studied and methodologies differ widely. Nevertheless we found two substances that were tested in two different trials but only one (*Mimosa pudica*) by two different investigators in different countries. They are not similar: in one it was tested in 3x and 6x and in the other using 6x, 6c, 9c, 12c, 30c prepared by different pharmaceutical companies. One used a parallel group and the other was an uncontrolled study. All in all we found a very different pattern of symptoms emerging in both reports (in the uncontrolled one six students had very severe reactions and most of the symptoms were related to digestive system; the other didn't report any withdrawal due to adverse reactions and compiled very few symptoms in the digestive area).

Table 5.5 compares the main characteristics of the best trials (only included in Classes I or II of EC and SMA indices).

Table 5.5 Characteristics of the best HPTs published in UK (1945–1995)

First author/year	*Medicine*	*Study design*	*Sample size*	*No. of controls*	*Incidence per volunteer*	*Adverse reaction report*	*Criteria to select symptoms*
Nagpaul, 1989	*Tarantula hispanica*	Parallel	28	8	19.25	no	Confirmation in other volunteers
Clover, 1980	*Pulsatilla*	Crossover	18	18	0	no	Intensity of the symptom + statistical analysis
Pratt, 1971	*Lycopodium Rhustoxico-dendron Spigelia Magnesia Phosphorica*	Parallel	103	52 (?)	0.2	no	Not stated
Walach, 1993	*Belladonna*	Crossover	45	45	0	yes (2%)	Statistical analysis

Outcome measures

Pathogenetic effects are traditionally collected in HPTs by diaries and 44% of the studies stated that a diary was used. Of these, 20% were semi-structured diaries suggesting only areas where symptoms could occur and 40% were open diaries.

Criteria for causality assessment

Eighty-four per cent of the reports did not state any criteria for deciding on which grounds the symptoms were considered to have a causal association with the tested medicine. In only one of the reports was there a list of six criteria used to select pathogenetic effects but the report did not explain how the criteria were applied to select the symptoms (28). This publication summarizes many of the criteria sparsely described in other papers and includes occurrence shortly after taking the medicine, intensity of the symptom, duration of the symptom, peculiarity of the symptom, occurrence of the symptom in other volunteers and modalities and concomitants associated with a symptom.

Safety

Adverse reactions were reported in 13 trials (19.4%) comprising 31 events and thus an overall incidence of adverse reactions of 4.8% (31/641). One author reported 22 adverse reactions after five uncontrolled trials. In the best trials the incidence of adverse reactions was 0.7% (1/134) and was similar to nocebo reactions. Both crossover trials showed a larger number of symptoms or changes under placebo compared to verum phases for some volunteers.

Discussion

A considerable number of HPTs have been conducted in the 50 years between 1945 and 1995. There is a great deal of variability in the studies in terms of the medicines tested, methodology, volunteers, sample size and outcome. This was reflected in great variability in the numbers, incidence and types of effects reported. There was a clear association between the methodological quality of the trial and the numbers of effects reported: better trials produced a lower incidence of pathogenetic effects (or none) compared to trials of poorer quality. Overall the analysis of reports revealed methodological shortcomings which, in our opinion seriously compromise the validity, reliability and clinical applicability of the results. It is not possible to reach a definite conclusion regarding the true effects of homoeopathic medicines in healthy volunteers because of differences in the trials and missing information in the reports. It is clear that bias varies widely between studies. Even if we take separately only the best trials we cannot accurately estimate the precision of the effect size or apply inferential statistics to analyse our data.

Several factors may account for the great variability in the results. Among others one can pinpoint the settings in which they were done, the lack of description of inclusion and exclusion criteria for volunteers, differences in study design and use of placebo, style of supervision and assumptions concerning attribution of symptoms to the medicine tested.

The identification and causal attribution of changes in healthy volunteers is very complex and may be influenced by a large number of factors. It is strongly dependent on individual awareness and past experiences. In the absence of adequate control, clinical studies can yield results favouring investigators' assumptions if the study is not properly controlled, context is also important (Green, 1964; Reidenberg and Lowenthal, 1968). The importance of conditioning was demonstrated in medical students in an experiment where students were conditioned to expect sedative or stimulant effects but received only placebo in blue or pink capsules. Volunteers' behaviour pattern has also been shown to influence the reporting of subjective symptoms after placebo (Drici *et al.*, 1995). Most of the HPTs reviewed here were done in the context of homoeopathic courses with students learning homoeopathy. In this situation two factors could bias the outcome towards increased reporting of symptoms: the students, believers in the system and the production, in the past, of valid symptoms from HPTs; and the coordinator expecting the students to give him useful information after testing the substance.

The definition of 'healthy' is also a problem. Joubert *et al.* (1975) showed that laboratory criteria of abnormality are unsuited to the purpose of selecting normal and abnormal volunteers. When they were stated, the major criterion for exclusion of non-healthy volunteers in our sample was clinical history. Yet there may be problems with this, the fluctuation of the occurrence of symptoms across time in apparently healthy people is well documented, particularly in placebo-controlled Phase 1 clinical trial reports (Sibille *et al.*, 1992; Rosenzweig *et al.*, 1993). This could account for incorrect attribution of symptoms as pathogenetic. It is impossible in the current state of knowledge to predict how many healthy volunteers might develop new symptoms or a recurrence of old symptoms in a given period of time. But the focus on self-observation and daily recording may result in an increased recall of changes during the experiment.

The use of weak and uncontrolled designs with multiple endpoints probably inflated the number of effects reported in the studies we reviewed. Only a small number (9) of trials described using a pre-observation period with or without placebo and they did not present the symptoms collected during this period and differences from the reported pathogenetic effects. As early as 1895 it was proposed that every HPT should be preceded by a pre-observation period to prepare the volunteer 'to pass judgement upon the pathogenetic value of the many manifestations that are likely to occur during the trial' (Medical Investigation Club of Baltimore, 1895). It is regrettable that this suggestion has not been more widely adopted.

The purpose of including a placebo group in many of these HPTs is not the same as in standard modern clinical trial designs. Normally, placebo is used to provide a statistical comparison with the outcome of the experimental group. To maximize statistical power, the placebo group should be approximately the same size as the active treatment group. If this method were applied in an HPT one would compare symptoms reported by volunteers on placebo and homoeopathic medicine. But, in many of the trials we examined, the intent behind the use of placebo was quite different: placebo was given to a small proportion of volunteers (typically 10–15%) in a parallel group design with the intention of ensuring that volunteers are truthful and take particular care in recording their symptoms (Sherr, 1994). As we have shown there was, at least in HPTs conducted in London in the 1950s and '60s, a progressive tendency to reduce and finally eliminate the use of placebo. The same tendency is seen in more recent investigations. But given Hahnemann's direction that investigators should select careful volunteers, placebo would be unnecessary if focusing the minds and ensuring the honesty of volunteers was the only reason for using it. This seems to be the line of thought which resulted in placebo control being described as a waste of time and volunteers.

However, the use of placebo symptoms purely for the purpose of quantitative statistical comparison seems to us too narrow. Both qualitative and quantitative evaluation is required if we are to understand what happens to healthy volunteers taking homoeopathic medicines compared to placebo in well-designed, rigorous HPTs.

Most of the HPTs published in the UK were conducted by a small number of investigators. The style of supervision and the judgement for the inclusion of pathogenetic effects could be, in an uncontrolled design, a powerful factor leading to over or under-inclusion of symptoms in the final publication. The incidence of reported adverse events was very variable; one supervisor reported a very high incidence, irrespective of the toxicity of the substance tested. Does this say something about the relationship of the supervisor with the volunteers (his students), or is it attributable to past experiences and expectations of the volunteers? At present one can only speculate. We can assume that homoeopaths expect useful information from HPTs. It may be that the personal beliefs of the supervisors and the pressure to present plenty of symptoms could lead to inclusion of large number of effects and discourage use of controls for comparison. The expectation of the homoeopathic practitioners of useful and peculiar symptoms after HPTs was well expressed by Templeton in his first published HPT (35): 'Now I can hear someone say, "Well that's not much of a proving. You have a few vague mentals more marked than anything else. Nothing here to cure cancer, duodenal ulcer, epilepsy".'

Publication bias cannot be excluded from playing a role in our findings. We did not investigate this matter further but one of the best reports – where the null hypothesis could not be statistically rejected – had its publication postponed for almost seven years 'in the hope of arranging further trials on the same model'. Taken together they raise the possibility of an inflation on the magnitude of effects in our sample due to non-publication of negative results.

Our results show a higher incidence of effects per volunteer when the methodological rigour of the trial is low. Taken as a whole, it appears that HPTs have hitherto greatly overestimated incidence of effects. From a theoretical perspective this is consistent with the flaws (from the perspective of modern methodological standards) in Hahnemann's original directions for conducting HPTs. These flaws have been discussed elsewhere (Dantas, 1996). The most important are: the absence or inadequacy of a control group, use of friends and 'believers' as volunteers, absent or inadequate masking of volunteers and/or investigators, excessively close supervision, absence of a pre-treatment 'run in' observation period, expectancy and conditioning effects and inclusion of non-healthy volunteers.

Our findings are also consistent with other studies of medical literature showing that estimates of treatment effects are exaggerated in trials of poor methodological quality (Schulz *et al.*, 1995).

These results are not dissimilar from other works reported in the medical literature. In the area of toxicology, for instance, Buckley and Smith (1996) showed that case series with more than seven cases provide the best available evidence to address the clinical and epidemiological problems of antihistamine poisoning. They also report that many textbooks still quote a review of antihistamine poisoning published in 1951, based on case reports. The quality of the data and conclusions are similar to our findings. In a study of RCTs published in UK public health journals, the authors found there was no detectable improvement in the quality of reports, despite the increase in the number of publications (Fahey *et al.*, 1995). The same applies to meta-analysis reports on analgesic interventions: 90% of the meta-analyses had methodological flaws limiting their validity (Jadad and McQuay, 1996).

Another issue is related to the rationale guiding HPTs. Substances investigated on the basis of rationales that do not comply with the principle of pathophysiological similarity were tested and yielded pathogenetic effects. It was surprising to find that most HPTs were done because of known properties of medicinal plants rather than toxic properties. Trials using substances with very low degree of toxicity in humans, sometimes selected on symbolic grounds ('Doctrine of Signatures' etc.), such as edible bird's nest, chocolate and human milk yielded a large number of effects. Analysis of the best reports shows that even randomized trials using comparison with placebo symptoms can yield a very large number of effects attributed to the medicine, if they rely only on the investigator's judgement with no statistical analysis or predefined criteria for symptom selection.

The use of quality indices to analyse published papers is controversial (Greenland, 1994; Olkin, 1994). For the sake of balance we used two indices based on different groups of parameters. The experimental control index was based on the assumption that randomization helps to reduce bias in clinical experiments; it combines this assumption with other features minimizing bias. On the other hand the SMA index was based on the two reviewers' overall impressions and ranking compared to other trials, after reading the report and completing the questionnaire. The moderate agreement observed between the two reviewers in this index shows this is prone to personal beliefs and knowledge of reviewers judging a report. On the other hand the moderate agreement between both indexes signals that one can reasonably accept our classification of scientific quality of the papers and its association with the number of findings claimed in the report.

The consistency of the effects across trials is another matter. Many investigators seemed to have taken for granted that every substance must elicit symptoms and for this reason felt it unnecessary to use placebo as a control or failed to include symptoms experienced by volunteers taking placebo. On the other hand the use of placebo exclusively for comparative statistical purpose excludes from consideration rare, idiosyncratic effects. Attempts by Martini in the 1930s to evaluate the occurrence of pathogenetic effects due to highly diluted substances in HPTs were, on the whole, negative and a critical reappraisal of his results shows that no definite conclusion can be drawn (Walach, 1991).

Inadequate use of control and failure to use placebo symptoms as a comparator leads to overestimation of pathogenetic effects. But the use of an exclusively quantitative statistical analysis probably leads to underestimation of pathogenetic effects. 'Rare, strange and peculiar' or idiosyncratic symptoms are believed to be of crucial importance in homoeopathic prescribing, yet they may occur in only a few or no volunteers in a small group. In an HPT of traditional parallel group design such idiosyncratic effects would be drowned in statistical 'noise' arising from spontaneous, incidental or irrelevant sources. The use of crossover designs is a possible solution, but there may be serious problems with order effects and treatment/period interactions ('carry-over effects'). It is also possible that it is the quality or character, rather than the quantity of symptoms, that is important. These problems have not yet been adequately addressed, the lessons that can be learnt from traditional randomized controlled trials in these areas are relatively few. In our view they are important areas for methodological development.

HPTs play various roles for homoeopathy. From an historical perspective they are powerful evidence of the experimental nature of homoeopathy since its inception. Their results have been disseminated and applied by homoeopathic practitioners worldwide. For some homoeopaths, HPTs are the basis of homoeopathy; others view them as marginal, a view that can be defended, since most of the homoeopathic materia medica is based on clinical indications gathered from prescribing homoeopathic remedies to patients. On the regulatory front attempts have been made to have HPTs required to license new homoeopathic products. Our results show the evidence for the occurrence of pathogenetic effects in HPTs is contaminated. There is at present no definitive answer, from a critical perspective, to the main question posed in HPTs, namely: do homoeopathic medicines in high dilution provoke changes in healthy volunteers? If appropriate and well-designed research gives a negative answer to this question, we should accept the role of HPTs as purely historical and expunge information deriving from them from the homoeopathic database. On the other hand if research shows that they can produce specific effects, but only in a minority of volunteers, we will need to re-study and reformulate the process used to get information from HPTs.

On the basis of these results we suggest developing and comparing a limited range of well controlled study designs, using homoeopathic medicines from sources of differing toxicity, preferably in 30cH dilution. Only by this means can the assumption generally held in homoeopathy, that homoeopathic medicines can elicit symptoms in healthy volunteers, be tested. The studies we reviewed claim, on average, that homoeopathic dilutions can elicit at least one symptom in 75% of volunteers. We are sceptical of this claim but if it is true then controlled studies with small sample sizes followed by at least four weeks of follow-up would be appropriate. The better designed studies among those we reviewed claimed a much lower incidence of effects, and sometimes no statistically significant quantitative difference between active and placebo treatment. If there is evidence that a small minority of volunteers manifest changes when using homoeopathic medicines compared to placebo (and there are findings in some of the better designed studies which suggest that this is the case) then we will require new designs, perhaps drawing on experience for the detection of type II, or idiosyncratic, adverse drug reactions.

In any case new HPTs should include a definition of a healthy volunteer for the purpose of the trial and an assessment of health status. They should use representative populations, methods designed to minimize bias and suggestion and the attribution of spontaneous or unrelated changes to the medicine, clear instructions for volunteers and supervisors, sensitive and valid outcomes measurements.

Physicians are obliged to follow ethical guidelines regarding experimentation in humans. The voluntary consent of the human subject was expressly required for experiments on human subjects in the Nuremberg Code (1947). This was again acknowledged in the Declaration of Helsinki, in particular for non-clinical biomedical research using healthy volunteers or patients for whom the experimental design is not related to their illness. It follows that it should be mandatory to get informed consent from all volunteers and to seek Ethics Committee approval for HPTs.

The quality of the publication of HPTs could be enhanced if editors of homoeopathic journals agreed on minimal requirements for reporting such trials. These should include adequate description of the setting and of the medicine tested (source, mode of preparation, posology), inclusion and exclusion criteria, withdrawals, demographic data, ethical approval, study design and criteria for selection of pathogenetic changes. Structured reporting of HPTs might also be helpful, allowing easy extraction of the main points.

Homoeopathy, folly or medicine? It is undoubtedly true that the HPT, when introduced by Hahnemann 200 years ago, was a revolutionary and genuinely experimental method, far ahead of its time. It has subsequently been developed by committed investigators. On the negative side, our systematic review has shown that some recent HPTs lack adequate control and analysis; the results of such studies are unreliable and maybe positively misleading and damaging to both homoeopathy and to patients.

As evidence for the efficacy of homoeopathy from controlled therapeutic trials accumulates, there is an increasing need to investigate and develop valid methodologies for the basic method of homoeopathy – the homoeopathic pathogenetic trial.

Acknowledgements

During the preparation of this paper the first author was supported by a Post-Doctoral Fellowship from CNPq (Conselho Nacional de Desenvolvimento Científico e Tecnológico do Brasil) but endorsement by this agency is not implied.

References

Altman, D. (1996) Better reporting of randomised controlled trials: the CONSORT statement. *BMJ*, **313**, 570–1.

Anello, C. and Fleiss, J.L. (1995) Exploratory or analytic meta-analysis: should we distinguish between them? *J. Clin. Epidemiol.*, **48**, 109–16.

Buckley, N.A. and Smith, A.J. (1996) Evidence-based medicine in toxicology: where is the evidence? *Lancet*, **347**, 1167–9.

Dantas, F. (1996) How can we get more reliable information from homoeopathic pathogenetic trials? A critique of 'provings'. *Br. Hom. J.*, **85**, 230–36.

Drici, M., Raybaud, F., De Lunardo, C., Iacono, P. and Gustovic, P. (1995) Influence of the behaviour pattern on the nocebo response of healthy volunteers. *Br. J. Clin. Pharmacol.*, **39**, 204–6.

Fahey, T., Hyde, C., Milne, R. and Thorogood, M. (1995) The type and quality of randomized controlled trials (RCTs) published in UK public health journals. *J. Publ. Hlth. Med.*, **17**, 469–74.

Green, D.M. (1964) Pre-existing conditions, placebo reactions and 'side effects'. *Ann. Int. Med.*, **60**, 255–65.

Greenland, S. (1994) Invited Commentary: A critical look at some popular meta-analytic methods. *Am. J. Epidemiol.*, **140**, 290–6.

Haehl, R. (1983) *Samuel Hahnemann: his life and work*, p. 103, v. 2. New Delhi: Jain.

Hahnemann, S. (1982; translated from the sixth German edition) *The Organon of Medicine*. Los Angeles: J.P. Tarcher.

Hahnemann, S. (1913; translated from the first German edition) *Organon of the Rational Art of Healing*. London; J.M.Dent & Sons Ltd.

Hahnemann, S. (1936) *Materia medica pura*, p. 19, v. 1. London; Homoeopathic Publishing Co.

Jadad, A.R. and McQuay, H.J. (1996) Meta-Analyses to evaluate analgesic interventions: a systematic qualitative review of their methodology. *J. Clin. Epidemiol.*, **49**, 235–43.

Joubert, P., Rivera-Calimlim, L. and Lasagna, L. (1975) The normal volunteer in clinical investigation: How rigid should selection criteria be? *Clin. Pharmacol. Ther.*, **17**, 253–7.

Medical Research Council (1948) Streptomycin treatment of pulmonary tuberculosis. *BMJ*, **ii**, 769–82.

Mulrow, C.D. (1987) The medical review article: State of the Science. *Ann. Intern. Med.*, **106**, 485–8.

Olkin, I. (1994) Invited Commentary: Re: 'A critical look at some popular meta-analytic methods'. *Am. J. Epidemiol.*, **140**, 297–9.

Reidenberg, M.M. and Lowenthal, D.T. (1968) Adverse nondrug reactions. *New Eng. J. Med.*, **279**, 678–9.

Rosenzweig, P., Brohier, S. and Zipfel, A. (1993) The placebo effect in healthy volunteers: influence of experimental conditions on the adverse events profile during phase I studies. *Clin. Pharmacol. Ther.*, **54**, 578–83.

Sherr, J. (1994) *The dynamics and methodology of homoeopathic proving*. West Malvern: Dynamis Books.

Sibille, M., Deigat, N., Olagnier, V., Durand, D.V. and Levrat, R. (1992) Adverse events in phase one studies: a study in 430 health volunteers. *Eur. J. Clin. Pharmacol.*, **42**, 389–93.

Schulz, K.F., Chalmers, I., Hayes, R.J. and Altman, D.G. (1995) Empirical evidence of bias: dimensions of methodological quality associated with estimates of treatment effects in controlled trials. *JAMA*, **273**, 408–12.

The Medical Investigation Club of Baltimore (1895) *A pathogenetic materia medica*. Philadelphia: Boericke & Tafel.

Walach, H. (1991) Research in Homoeopathy in Germany during the Thirties: Inquiry by the Reichsgesundheitsamt 1936–1939, the remedy proving by Martini. *Berlin J. Research Hom.*, **1**, 325–38.

Notes

See superscript numbers in text.

1 Hahnemann used the word 'prüfung' when referring to homoeopathic trials in healthy volunteers. This word is normally translated into modern medical English as 'trial'. According to the ninth edition of *The Concise Oxford Dictionary* (COD), to prove has an 'archaic meaning – no longer in ordinary use, though retained for special purposes – of test the qualities of, *try'*. Nowadays to prove – from the Latin *probare* – has the main meaning of test, approve, demonstrate the truth of by evidence or argument (COD). *The New Shorter Oxford English Dictionary* teaches that to prove started to be used between 1830 and 1869 with a new principal sense of 'find out by experience, experience, suffer'. The word 'proving' is not separately cited in the COD.

2 HPTs in animals were excluded from our study. There are a few references on such studies in the homoeopathic literature. In France O.A. Julian did a trial to compare the effects of reserpine in rats, guinea-pigs and humans (*Cahiers de Biotherapie* (1967) **16**, 231–6).

3 We decided to exclude trials using exclusively mother tinctures or undiluted/unpotentized substances on the basis of their differential nature from the properly homoeopathic medicines. However it is important to acknowledge that Hahnemann used these substances to do pathogenetic trials in the beginning of homoeopathy but later on he moved to use only very diluted homoeopathic medicines (mostly 30C). Based on this criteria only one trial was excluded.

4 This is a conservative approximation as some substances were tested in the same volunteers in three different terms and there was crossover of volunteers using placebo or verum.

5 In two reports (3 and 45) there was no specific pathogenetic effect reported. However both trials analysed data using statistical techniques. In one a significant difference ($p<0.05$) was noticed between the number of symptoms experienced by 13 volunteers when taking verum and placebo; in Study 3 single case differences between phases were not calculated and the necessary data were not published.

List of included studies

See numbers in parenthesis in text.

1 Chakravarty, B.N. (1982) Solar eclipse ray. Proceedings of the 35th Liga Medica Homoeopathica Internationalis Congress, 1982; Sussex (UK): LMHI. pp. 392–7.
2 Chand, D.H. (1982) Cassia sophera. Proceedings of the 35th Liga Medica Homoeopathica Internationalis Congress, 1982; Sussex (UK): LMHI. pp. 381–6.
3 Clover, A.M., Jenkins S., Campbell, A.C. and Jenkins, M.D. (1980) Report on a proving of Pulsatilla 3x. *Br. Hom. J.,* **69**, 134–47.
4 Daws, J. and Scriven, D. (1992) *The making and proving of Sol Britannic*. Tunbridge Wells: Helios.
5 Engel, P.B. (1975) A proving of Nidus edulis. *Br. Hom. J.,* **64**, 224–30.
6 Houghton, J. and Halahan, E. (1995) *The homoeopathic proving of Lac humanum*. Authors' edition.
7 Julian, O. (1964) Pathogenesis of Nepenthes. *Br. Hom. J.,* **53**, 259–66.
8 Julian, O.A. (1983) Pathogenesis of Platinum 1980. *Br. Hom. J.,* **72**, 31–50.
9 Kenyon, J.D., Wheeler, C.E. and Woods, H.F. (1947) Drug Proving Committee. *Br. Hom. J.,* **37**, 64–6.
10 McIvor, E.G. (1980) Phormium tenax – a proving. *Br. Hom. J.,* **69**, 26–32.
11 McIvor, E.G. (1975) Gingko biloba – a proving. *Br. Hom. J.,* **64**, 105–6.
12 Nagpaul, V.M., Dhawan, I.M., Vichitra, A.K. and Rastogi, D.P. (1989) Tarentula hispanica – a reproving. *Br. Hom. J.,* **78**, 19–26.
13 O'Hanlon, M. (1952) A short proving of Strophantus Sarmentosus. *Br. Hom. J.,* **42**, 13–15.
14 Pai, P.N. (1965) A proving of Chlorpromazine. *Br. Hom. J.,* **54**, 102–4.
15 Pai, P.N. (1967) A proving of Texanus toxin. *Br. Hom. J.,* **56**, 94–100.
16 Pratt, N.J. (1971) Double blind proving trial by medical students. *Br. Hom. J.,* **60**, 41–3.
17 Raeside, J.R. (1959) A proving of Hydrophis Cyanocinctus. *Br. Hom. J.,* **48,** 196–214.
18 Raeside, J.R. (1960) A proving of Triosteum perfoliatum. *Br. Hom. J.,* **49**, 269–78.
19 Raeside, J.R. (1961) Report on a proving of Selenium. *Br. Hom. J.,* **50**, 215–25.
20 Raeside, J.R. (1962) A proving of Venus mercenaria. *Br. Hom. J.,* **51**, 200–6.
21 Raeside, J.R. (1964) A proving of Hirudo medicinalis. *Br. Hom. J.,* **53**, 22–30.
22 Raeside, J.R. (1965) A proving of Esponjilla (Luffa operculata). *Br. Hom. J.,* **54**, 36–44.
23 Raeside, J.R. (1966) A proving of Mandragora Officinarum. *Br. Hom. J.,* **55**, 68–75.
24 Raeside, J.R. (1967) A proving of Colchicum autumnale. *Br. Hom. J.,* **56**, 86–93.
25 Raeside, J.R. (1968) A proving of Tellurium. *Br. Hom. J.,* **57**, 216–20.
26 Raeside, J.R. (1969) A proving of Flor de Piedra (Lophophytum leandri). *Br. Hom. J.,* **58**, 240–6.
27 Raeside, J.R. (1971) A proving of Mimosa pudica. *Br. Hom. J.,* **60**, 97–104.
28 Riley, D. (1995) Proving report – Veronica officinalis. *Br. Hom. J.,* **84**, 144–8.
29 Sankaran, P. (1970) Atrax robustus, a proving. *Br. Hom. J.,* **59**, 44–5.
30 Sankaran, P. (1970) A proving of Mimosa pudica. *Br. Hom. J.,* **59**, 42–3.
31 Sherr, J. (1985) *The homoeopathic proving of Scorpion*. Tiverton: The Society of Homoeopaths.
32 Sherr, J. (1993) *The homeopathic proving of Chocolate*. Northampton: Dynamis School for Advanced Homoeopathic Studies.
33 Sherr, J. (1992) *The homeopathic proving of Hydrogen*. Northampton: Dynamis School of Homoeopathy.
34 Smith, T. (1979) A proving of Kali carb. *Br. Hom. J.,* **68**, 88–92.
35 Templeton, W.L. (1949) Cadmium metallicum. *Br. Hom. J.,* **39**, 60–4.
36 Templeton, W.L. (1949) Provings of Alloxan. *Br. Hom. J.,* **39**, 246–81.
37 Templeton, W.L. (1951) A third proving of alloxan. *Br. Hom. J.,* **41**, 111–19.
38 Templeton, W.L. (1952) Proving of Strophantus Sarmentosus. *Br. Hom. J.,* **42**, 4–12.
39 Templeton, W.L. (1953) Report on Beryllium provings. *Br. Hom. J.,* **43**, 78–84.

40 Templeton, W.L. (1954) Provings of Carcinosin. *Br. Hom. J.,* **44**, 108–15.
41 Templeton, W.L. (1956) Provings of Cortisone and ACTH. *Br. Hom. J.,* **45**, 89–97.
42 Templeton, W.L. (1956) Report on Rauwolfia serpentina. *Br. Hom. J.,* **45**, 155–66.
43 Vakil, AE, Nanabhai, A.S. and Vakil, Y.E. (1989) A study of Iris Versicolor 3c. *Br. Hom. J.,* **78**, 15–18.
44 Vakil, A.E., Vakil, V.E. and Nanabhal, A.S. (1988) Iodum. *Br. Hom. J.,* **77**, 152–4.
45 Walach, H. (1993) Does a highly diluted homoeopathic act as a placebo in healthy volunteers? Experimental Study of Belladonna 30C in double-blind crossover design – a pilot study. *J. Psychosomatic Res.,* **37**, 851–60.

Part III

Clinical Aspects: Efficiency and Safety

Chapter 6

Overviews and meta-analyses of controlled clinical trials of homoeopathy

*Klaus Linde, Nicola Clausius, Gilbert Ramirez, Dieter Melchart, Florian Eitel, Larry V. Hedges and Wayne B. Jonas**

Introduction

Although relevant progress has been made in the last few years, the discussion related to homoeopathy is still fundamental and the positions are very strong. Is homoeopathy madness or medicine? On the level of clinical research, 'madness' could be operationalized by the hypothesis all clinical effects of homoeopathy (if there are any) are due to placebo and 'medicine' by the hypothesis that homoeopathy is in general more than placebo. On a broader scientific level madness would also encompass that homoeopathy is irrational while to be considered scientific medicine, homoeopathy should be both rational and more effective than placebo.

It is clear that these positions are very far apart, but also that they leave important questions uncovered: for example, even if homoeopathy is in some cases more than a placebo, does this mean that it is an effective therapy in general or in a specific condition? Or, even if homoeopathy is not more than a placebo, is it an especially effective placebo? This chapter will, however, be restricted to investigating whether homoeopathy is 'madness or medicine' with respect to clinical research.

Overviews of clinical trials of homoeopathy

Our first step in 1992/1993 was to investigate existing overviews of clinical trials of homoeopathy (Linde *et al.*, 1994). We tried to identify as many overviews as possible by searching electronic as well as other databases, by contacting researchers in the field and manufacturers of homoeopathic preparations, and by checking the references in articles thus obtained for other relevant references. In order to be included for further analysis, review articles had to

* The views, opinions and assertions expressed in this article are those of the authors and do not reflect official policy of the National Institutes of Health, the Department of Health and Human Services, or the US Government.

be published after 1986 and reference more than 10 clinical trials comparing a homoeopathic intervention with a control intervention (in 1991 at least 107 such trials were available). From the review articles meeting the inclusion criteria we extracted the numbers of primary studies summarized, studies of individualized homoeopathy, studies with 'positive' or 'negative' results, and reviewers' conclusions. The scientific validity of the overviews was assessed according to predefined criteria (specification of the research question, methods of literature searching, inclusion/exclusion criteria, assessment of the primary studies according to predefined criteria, proportion of studies identified, and methods used for summarizing study results).

We identified 41 papers which could be classified as review papers dealing with clinical research. Only nine of these fully referenced more than ten controlled clinical trials and only two could be classified as systematic reviews (i.e. reviews performed according to predefined explicit methods) (Hill and Doyon, 1990; Kleijnen, Knipschild and ter Riet, 1991).

Hill and Doyon (1990) included 40 randomized trials in their review. In 19 trials the results were classified as being in favour of homoeopathy, 19 trials were classified as showing no efficacy and two trials were not assessable. Hill and Doyon concluded that the proof for the efficacy of homoeopathic medicines is inadequate.

Kleijnen *et al.* (1991) identified 107 controlled clinical trials, 68 of which were randomized. In 81 trials, the results with respect to homoeopathy were 'positive', in 24 they were 'negative' and two trials were not assessable. The methodological quality of the trials was assessed according to a list of predefined criteria and quantified by a scoring system. Although most of the trials were of low methodological quality, there were several high quality trials. Furthermore, the number of these high quality trials with 'positive' results clearly exceeded that of those with 'negative' results. Kleijnen *et al.* concluded that on the basis of the existing evidence they would be ready to accept that homoeopathy can be efficacious if only the mechanism of action would be more plausible.

Further comparison of the two systematic reviews revealed more disagreements. Among the 40 trials included by Hill and Doyon, seven were rated as non-randomized by Kleijnen and colleagues, and two trials explicitly excluded by Hill and Doyon for not being truly randomized were classified as randomized by Kleijnen and colleagues. Among the 19 studies rated as 'negative' by Hill and Doyon, seven were counted 'positive' by the other reviewers. This was due to a different method of categorizing study results.

While the review by Hill and Doyon received relatively little attention outside of France (it was published in a French journal), the comprehensive overview of Kleijnen *et al.* published in the *British Medical Journal* became the paper of reference. Despite the high quality of this overview in comparison to most overviews in medicine, it was criticized for two shortcomings, in particular:

1 In the quality assessment, a crucial issue of methodological quality – handling of drop-outs/withdrawals – was not included;
2 The method of categorizing results into 'positive' and 'negative' is open to bias and leading statisticians do not recommend this method.

Objective and methods of a new systematic review

Given these shortcomings and the publication of a relevant number of new controlled trials since 1991, we decided to do a new overview. The objective was to investigate in more detail the hypothesis that 'all clinical effects of homoeopathy are due to placebo'. Two approaches were chosen to investigate this hypothesis. The primary approach was to quantitatively summarize the effect size observed with homoeopathic remedies, compared with placebo in all randomized, double-blind, placebo-controlled clinical trials reported up to October 1995 (overall comparison test). The second approach was to see if any effect comparison between homoeopathy and placebo is independently reproducible in a single medical condition using a single homoeopathic strategy, remedy, population and outcome measure (reproducibility test). Using these two approaches gives both an overall estimate of effect differences and an assessment of the reproducibility of those effects in specific clinical conditions.

Inclusion/exclusion criteria

The following inclusion criteria were defined *a priori*:

1 study subjects had to be humans;
2 there had to be either an explicit statement that the study was randomized (including forms of quasi-randomization such as alternation, etc.) or an explicit statement that the trial was double-blind (therapist and patient) which makes some sort of random or quasi-random allocation likely;
3 the test intervention had to be a strategy involving the application of a homoeopathically prepared remedy;
4 the control intervention had to be placebo;
5 the trial had to be on the treatment or prevention of pathologic conditions or symptoms.

We excluded:

1 homoeopathic drug provings (a type of homoeopathic investigation aimed to collect information on symptoms provoked by the remedy in healthy volunteers);
2 trials on healthy volunteers which did not investigate the prevention or treatment of pathologic symptoms, but only the modification of physiological parameters;
3 single-case experiments.

Search strategy

The following sources were used to search for eligible trials: the review by Kleijnen, Knipschild and ter Riet (1991); Medline and Embase databases; contacts with researchers and manufacturers; congress proceedings and homoeopathic journals; the complementary medicine databases CISCOM (RCCM, London), AMED (British Library) and IDAG (Amersfoor). All searches were performed in 1994 and 1995; additional online searches in Embase and Medline were performed for the period 1989 to 1994.

Data extraction and assessment of methodological quality

In a first phase a large amount of information on source characteristics, design, patients, interventions, outcomes and results was extracted using specially developed data extraction forms. All test interventions were classified as individualized homoeopathy, formula/clinical homoeopathy, isopathy or use of complex preparations.

After having screened the trials the following preference-based strategy for extracting trial results for meta-analysis was used by two independent reviewers.

- First preference (p1): if available, data on a predefined main outcome measure (or the outcome on which a sample size calculation was performed) were extracted.
- Second preference (p2): if p1 data were not available, data on patients' global assessments were extracted.
- Third preference (p3): if p1 and p2 data were not available, data on physicians' global assessments were extracted.
- Fourth preference (p4): if p1, p2, and p3 data were not available, data for the clinically most important outcome measure (e.g. duration of illness in trials on treatment of upper respiratory tract infections) were extracted if possible.

If there were multiple outcome measures, each with sufficient data reported (making a reasonable choice impossible), each outcome was allocated a number and a dice was thrown to determine what outcome to use. Trials which did not present sufficient data were excluded from meta-analysis.

Aspects of methodological quality of primary studies were assessed independently by two reviewers in an open fashion using two scales:

1. A scale developed and validated by Jadad *et al.* (1996), which includes three items with a maximum score of five points (two points each for random allocation and blinding, one point for description of drop-outs and withdrawals);
2. A scale developed by one of the reviewers which has seven items and a maximum of seven score points (two items each on random allocation and blinding, one item each on baseline comparability, handling of withdrawals and inferential statistics; one point for each item).

The latter scale has already been used in two other areas of complementary medicine (Linde *et al.*, 1996a, b). Disagreements were discussed and a final score was agreed upon.

Meta-analysis

For all trials presenting sufficient data, odds ratios and 95 per cent confidence intervals were calculated. Continuous outcome data were transformed to odds ratios using a relation by Hasselblad and Hedges (1995). A pooled effect size estimate was calculated for the overall comparison (using the random effects model) and for several predefined sensitivity and subgroup analyses.

Preliminary results and discussion

A total of 186 controlled trials in humans were identified (excluding provings). A placebo group was included in 133 clinical trials, but 14 of these were not randomized and/or double blind. Of the 119 placebo-controlled, randomized and/or double-blind clinical trials, 89 presented sufficient data for meta-analysis. The methodology of about two-thirds of the trials is weak, while about 10 per cent of the trials have excellent methodology. Preliminary analyses indicate that the available trials do not support the hypothesis that all clinical effects of homoeopathic interventions can be attributed to placebo. The sensitivity and subgroup analyses confirm these results. On the other hand, there is a lack of independent replications showing convincingly an effect of a defined homoeopathic intervention in a single condition. If these results are confirmed in final analyses it has to be concluded that either homoeopathic interventions have an effect over placebo, huge biases are present in the data-set available or that randomized, placebo-controlled clinical trials tend to produce false-positive results (see also Reilly *et al.*, 1994).

Performing further trials in new study models does not seem to be a useful approach to finally determining if all effects of homoeopathy are due to placebo. Independent replications of existing trials could instead provide relevant new evidence. However, as most of the study models investigated hardly represent the homoeopathic treatment provided in daily practice, 'negative' results would be unlikely to have relevant practical implications even for those homoeopathic practitioners who are open to controlled trials.

It seems questionable if a research strategy dealing almost exclusively with a 'general placebo question' is adequate to provide useful answers for clinical decision-making. In our opinion, it is mandatory to collect reliable information on patient characteristics, interventions, outcomes and success rates under 'real life' conditions and with a variety of study designs. Such data could provide a rational basis for planning effective and efficient randomized trials in future.

Acknowledgements

Part of this work is performed within the MD of Nicola Clausius, currently under preparation at the Medical Faculty of the Ludwig-Maximilians-University Munich, under the supervision of Prof. F. Eitel and was partially supported by a grant from the Karl and Veronica Carstens Foundation (Essen, Germany).

References

Hasselblad, V. and Hedges, L.V. (1995) Meta-analysis of diagnostic and screening tests. *Psycholog. Bull.*, **117**, 167–78.

Hill, C. and Doyon, F. (1990) Review of randomized trials of homoeopathy. *Rev. Epidemiol. Santé Publ.*, **38**, 139–47.

Jadad, A.R., Moore, R.A., Carrol, D., Jenkinson, C., Reynolds, D.J.M., Gavaghan, D.J. and McQuay, H.J. (1996) Assessing the quality of reports of randomized clinical trials: is blinding necessary? *Contr. Clin. Trials*, **17**, 1–12.

Kleijnen, J., Knipschild, P. and ter Riet, G. (1991) Clinical trials of Homoeopathy. *Br. Med. J.*, **302**, 316–23.

Linde, K., Melchart, D., Brandmaier, R. and Eitel, F. (1994) Übersichtsarbeiten – Das Beispiel Homöopathie. *Dt Ärzteblatt*, **91**, A108–12.

Linde, K., Ramirez, G, Mulrow, C.D., Pauls, A., Weidenhammeer, W. and Melchart, D. (1996a) St John's wort for depression – an overview and meta-analysis of randomized clinical trials. *Br. Med. J.*, **313**, 253–8.

Linde, K., Worku, F., Stör, W. *et al.* (1996b) Randomized clinical trials of acupuncture for asthma – a systematic review. *Forsch. Komplementärmed.*, **3**, 148–55.

Reilly, D., Taylor, M.A., Beattie, N. *et al.* (1994) Is evidence for homoeopathy reproducible? *Lancet*, **344**, 1601–6.

Chapter 7

Placebo effects

Edzard Ernst

Introduction

'Placebos have doubtless been used for centuries by wise physicians as well as by quacks' (Beecher, 1955). With this introductory sentence to his influential article, Beecher set the scene for a discussion that continued throughout the 1960s and has recently come to life again. While some medical researchers today may be suffering from 'placebo mania' (Rothman, 1996) most clinicians continue to be afflicted by 'placebo phobia'. For physicians in any type of medicine, the subject 'provokes a shudder of discomfort like a cold hand in the dark' (Wall, 1992).

In complementary medicine the 'aura of quackery' (Wall, 1992) linked to any discussion of the placebo effect is, for many, too close for comfort. In homoeopathy, the issue may be even more complex than in other types of medicine (Davidson, 1996): homoeopathy, it is often claimed, works through enhancing the self-healing processes; to some this could mean that homoeopathy simply aims to maximize the placebo response.

This chapter will briefly review the subject of placebo effects, focusing on aspects relevant in relation to homoeopathy. It is aimed at de-mystifying the topic and clarifying some of the confusion that often seems to exist (Melchart, 1996).

Definition

There are almost as many definitions of 'placebo' as groups researching the matter. Many of these definitions are not helpful. Gotzsche has recently published definitions which are both pragmatic and valuable (1994): 'The placebo effect is the difference in outcome between a placebo treated group and an untreated control group in an unbiased experiment'. The definition reflects the impossibility of defining the placebo effect in a given individual. In single cases, biases of various types cannot be excluded and therefore a definition will always be problematic. Gotzsche also tried to define a placebo as 'an intervention which is believed to lack a specific effect on the disease in question' but later discarded this definition because of the impossibility in defining what constitutes a specific effect (Gotzsche, 1994).

Perhaps the most generally accepted definition of a placebo is the well seasoned one of Shapiro and Morris who described placebo as 'any therapy or component of therapy that is used for its non-specific psychological or psychophysiological effect, or for its presumed specific effect, but is without specific activity for the condition being treated' (Shapiro and Morris, 1978). Again this runs into the difficulty of differentiating between specific and non-specific effects. Grünbaum therefore proposed a solution whereby a distinction between characteristic and incidental elements of the placebo effect should be distinguished instead (Grünbaum, 1986). This definition, however, collapses as soon as one considers physiological therapies.

A disarmingly simple definition was recently offered by Oh: '[Placebo] . . . is the form of a treatment without its substance' (Oh, 1994). This is pragmatic, yet it might not be applicable to all areas of medical treatment (particularly not to homoeopathy) and is too simplistic for others.

Realizing the considerable difficulties in defining 'placebo', some have suggested that the concept has outlived its usefulness altogether (Kirsch, 1986; Omer and London, 1989; Richardson, 1989). A way out of this dilemma could be to use placebo effects synonymously with non-specific effects and, in turn, differentiate these into 'physician attention, interest and concern in a healing setting; patient and physician expectations of treatment effects; the reputation, expense and impressiveness of the treatment; and characteristics of the setting that influence patients to report improvement' (Turner *et al.*, 1994).

Three other terms also deserve a brief mention. *Pseudo-placebos* are defined as interventions which are active in principle but not for the condition that is being treated (Ernst, 1992). They are popular in clinical practice (e.g. a vitamin prescribed to a patient complaining about chronic insomnia) because they overcome some of the logistic and ethical problems of deliberate placebo use (e.g. the deception of the patient is perceived as less when an active drug is prescribed). *Super-placebo* is a term coined by the author (Ernst, 1992). It refers to a treatment that is, in fact, a placebo but neither the prescriber nor the patient is aware of the lack of specific effects. Examples of super-placebos are treatments that have been used at a time when they were thought to work but later found to be ineffective. The placebo effect may be particularly powerful under such conditions hence the term super-placebo. The *Hawthorne effect* describes the tendency for people to change their behaviour because they are the target of special interest and attention. It may have the opposite direction to the placebo effect (Bouchet, Guillemin and Briacon, 1996).

Does the placebo effect really exist?

Recently, the very existence of placebo phenomena has been questioned (Kienle, 1995). This was done essentially on the basis of a re-analysis of the Beecher paper (Beecher, 1955). Kienle found that the studies quoted by Beecher do not provide unequivocal proof of the existence of placebo effects. This may well be true, however, it does not provide a sufficient basis for negating the placebo effect altogether.

Generally speaking, there are several reasons for changes in any given clinical condition: the natural history of the disease; specific effects of a treatment; non-specific effects (see above) and artefacts such as regression towards the mean (e.g. Bouchet, Guillemin and Briacon, 1996). In order to be sure that a 'perceived placebo effect' is a 'true placebo effect', it is not enough to observe changes within a placebo-treated group of patients and equate them with the placebo response. An untreated control group is needed in order to differentiate non-specific effects from the other above-mentioned factors (see also the definition by Gotzsche quoted above). There are few studies which were conducted with both a placebo and an untreated control group. The ones that exist have been analysed recently (Ernst and Resch, 1995a). This analysis shows that true placebo effects of variable size do unquestionably exist.

Most studies fail to differentiate between 'perceived' and 'true placebo effects'. Therefore the following discussion will, for simplicity, also equate the two.

Myths about placebo effects

Only 'imagined' complaints respond to placebo

The opinion that one can differentiate between 'true' and 'imagined' disease by administering a placebo and observing who responds is widespread (Ernst and Abbot, in press) but cruelly wrong. The fact is that hypochondriacs, depressives, individuals with somatic pain and virtually all other groups of patients can respond to placebo (Wall, 1992; Grünbaum, 1986; Richardson, 1989; Turner *et al.*, 1994; Kienle, 1995). To judge a patient on his/her placebo response would be to gravely misjudge these individuals.

A distinct responder personality exists

There has been a considerable amount of research on this topic; much of it has been contradictory. On balance, however, the (best) evidence suggests that a responder personality cannot be differentiated from a non-responder personality. If a difference exists, the nature of this difference has not yet been identified (Richardson, 1994). A recent trial of homoeopathy confirmed this inadvertently (Lepaisart, 1995). All patients were treated with placebo during a run-in phase and the 22 per cent who showed a response were excluded from the trial proper with a view to subsequently dealing exclusively with placebo non-responders. The trialists, however, were surprised to find that in the subsequent phase where one subgroup was treated with verum and the other with placebo, 75 per cent of those receiving placebo responded positively to it. This exemplifies that an individual who is a non-responder today can become a responder tomorrow for no apparent reason.

Only subjective variables can be altered

Often it is assumed that placebos only affect parameters that cannot be quantified objectively. This notion is clearly wrong (e.g. Ernst, 1992). On the contrary, the number and type of variables responsive to placebo seem to be limitless. Certainly objective and somatic variables are amongst them – even the concentration of constituents in patients' blood can be affected by placebos (e.g. Hashish, Feinman and Harvey, 1988; Ernst, 1992; Turner *et al.*, 1994; Richardson, 1994; Lepaisart, 1995).

The effect size is around 35 per cent

This myth can be traced back to Beecher (1955) who showed that in the 15 studies he reviewed an average of 35 per cent of the patients responded to placebo. This led to the misunderstanding that the size of the placebo effect is a constant of 35 per cent. The truth is that, depending on the boundary conditions, the placebo effect can vary from 0 to 100 per cent (e.g. Liberman, 1964; Richardson, 1994).

Placebo is the same as no therapy

The confusion regarding the terminology is Babylonian. Many authors equate giving a placebo to patients with doing nothing at all (Ernst and Resch, 1995b); this would be the same as negating the placebo phenomenon altogether (see above). However, most authors who equate placebos with no treatment do not want to make this point; quite simply, they are victims of confusion and sloppy thinking (Ernst and Resch, 1995b).

Placebo effects are always mild

This may be true for most cases, yet as a generalization this notion does not hold true. The most dramatic example of this may be that of Voodoo deaths (Ernst, 1996). Theoretically placebo effects can be stronger than those of active, demonstrably effective medication given for the same condition (Figure 7.1).

Placebo effects are always positive

Negative effects of placebo (nocebo effects) can be demonstrated in virtually every placebo-controlled trial. They may affect as many as 40 per cent of patients taking placebos (Tangrea, Adrianza and Helsel, 1994). A most curious and incompletely understood phenomenon is the fact that nocebo effects often mimic the nature of the side-effects of the active treatment in controlled trials (Cromie, 1963). By re-analysing recently published data (Freedman, 1995), this can easily be shown graphically (Figure 7.2). The most frequently reported nocebo effects are headache, drowsiness, tiredness, dizziness, nausea, pain and insomnia (Rosenzweig, Brochier and Zipfel, 1993).

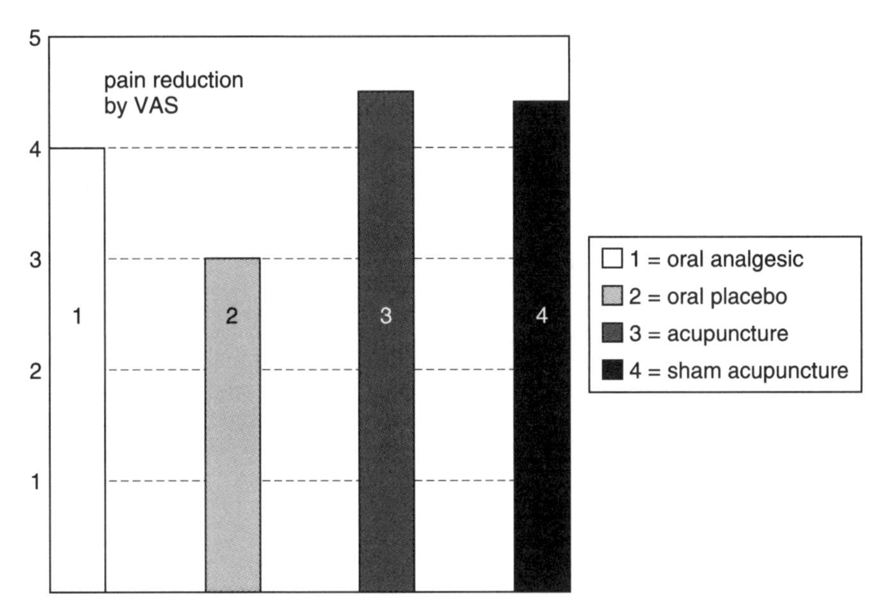

Figure 7.1 Example of a placebo effect being stronger than the effect of active medication. An example of a four-armed study in pain treatment. Although Treatment 1 could be significantly superior to 2, and Treatment 3 no different from 4, sham acupuncture could be significantly more effective than oral analgesic.

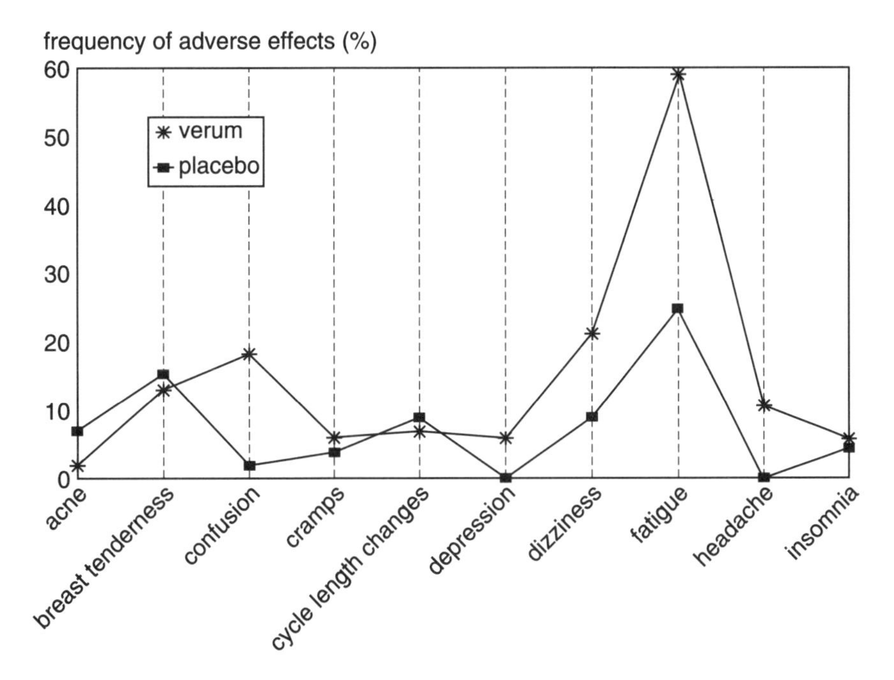

Figure 7.2 Nocebo effects. Adverse effects encountered in randomized, controlled trials on premenstrual syndrome.

Placebo effects are short-lasting

There is little research regarding the duration of placebo effects as most studies involve only short-term observations. The notion that long-term placebo responses do not exist, however, seems to be wrong (e.g. Ross and Olson, 1982). More work is needed to clarify this issue.

Animals do not respond to placebos

Most people who care for pets will observe that animals respond to care and concern, i.e. to non-specific effects, yet animals do not *know* they are receiving a medical intervention in the same way humans do. Pavlov's experiments are a good example of expectations having physiological effects on animals. Thus the argument 'homoeopathy works in animals and therefore cannot possibly be a placebo' is weak.

Mode of action

In his comprehensive overview, Richardson (1994) lists the following potential mechanisms of the placebo effect: operant conditioning, classical conditioning, guilt reduction, transference, suggestion, persuasion, role demands, hope, faith, labelling, selective symptom monitoring, misattribution, cognitive dissonance, control theory, anxiety reduction, expectancy effects, endorphin release and a variety of design and measurement artefacts. Most of these are based on little more than speculation. Some experimental evidence exists for the concepts of expectancy effects, cognitive dissonance, conditioning, anxiety reduction and endorphin release (Richardson, 1994). Recent evidence suggests an inhibitory role of cholecystokinin in the placebo response, implying a more complex biology of placebo (Benedetti, 1996). In each case, however, such findings are disputed. At present, therefore, the only conclusion that can be drawn is that the mode(s) of action of placebos is (are) not known.

Determinants

If we accept that the placebo response can vary from 0 to 100% (see above), it would be highly desirable to identify the factors that render one placebo more powerful than another. To date, these factors are also largely speculative.

Invasiveness of intervention

It has been said that surgery is associated with the most powerful placebo effect of all medical interventions. Almost 100% of patients submitted to 'sham-surgery' (skin incisions without an actual operation) show a response (Cobb *et al.*, 1959; Dimond, Kittle and Cockett, 1960). Similarly, placebo injections provoke stronger reactions than placebo pills (Carne, 1961; Grenfell, Briggs and Holland, 1961). Invasiveness, discomfort or pain experienced by the patient could therefore be an important factor.

The 'magic' of the intervention

This could be either a flavour of exoticism which surrounds therapies such as acupuncture or the magic of the 'high tech' or the unusual (e.g. individualization of homoeopathic treatment). Acupuncture is certainly associated with powerful placebo effects (Taub *et al.*, 1979), as are interventions using sophisticated equipment (Schwitzgebel and Traugott, 1968; Wickramasekera, 1977; Langley and Sheppeard, 1987). One might also assume that the degree of plausibility of an intervention could play a role, e.g. for someone who thinks that an imbalance of Yin and Yang causes disease, acupuncture might be associated with a particularly powerful placebo effect.

The therapist

Certain characteristics of the physician or therapist seem to induce stronger than average placebo responses. The status of the professional (Liberman, 1961; Lesse, 1962; Shapiro, 1964), his or her confidence in the treatment (Uhlenhuth *et al.*, 1959), and the amount of empathy shown could all play a role (Thomas, 1987). The information transmitted to the patient about the disease could be another determinant (Kaplan, Greenfield and Ware, 1989) and the therapist's expectations also seem to be important (Shapiro *et al.*, 1954; Gracely *et al.*, 1985).

The time factor

Although hard evidence is lacking, it seems conceivable that a long patient/doctor encounter might lead to stronger placebo effects than a short encounter. The time factor might work indirectly by increasing trust, expectation, etc. For homoeopathy it may be of particular relevance; on average a patient's first consultation with a homoeopathic practitioner lasts several times longer than one with a general practitioner (Fulder and Munro, 1985).

The patient

Patient expectation could be one of the strongest determinants of the placebo response. Experimental data show that this factor positively correlates with the observed outcome (e.g. Sternbach, 1964; Luparello *et al.*, 1970). The general attitude of the patient towards the doctor/therapist is likely to exert a similar influence and patient involvement with the therapy could be another factor. We have shown that administration of a topical placebo involving the patient in his/her treatment can lead to more powerful effects than the oral administration of placebo (Saradeth, Resch and Ernst, 1994).

The nature of the complaint

It would seem logical to assume that some conditions respond better to placebo than do others (Table 7.1). Much of the research on placebo has been conducted in conditions characterized by pain. We know that most other complaints and symptoms also respond to placebo. It would be valuable to re-address the question in a systematic way to determine whether some conditions are inherently more 'placebo prone' than others.

Table 7.1 Conditions that seem to be associated with a high (>30%) placebo-response rate

Conditions	*% of patients responding to placebo*
Headaches	62
Rheumatic conditions	49
Common colds	45
Gastrointestinal symptoms	38
Neuroses	34
Migraine	32

(Data from Janke, 1967)

The therapeutic setting

In a recent study, the therapeutic setting was the only significant predictor for nocebo effects (Tangrea, Adrianza and Helsel, 1994). The authors were unable to determine more precisely what the important characteristics of the setting were. It is possible that a formal clinical setting is more effective than an informal one. 'White coat hypertension' (the rise in blood pressure in the presence of a white-coated professional) could be a good example of this phenomenon.

From the above discussion, it follows that the culture surrounding homoeopathy is such that large placebo effects might be expected. For example, there is a comparatively long, detailed and empathic patient–therapist encounter, an exotic history and aura surrounding the therapy, a confidence in efficacy on the part of the therapist, a high expectation of (and cost for) the patient, etc. In a recent trial of homoeopathy versus placebo in 132 individuals with pollinosis, Wiesenauer and Lüdtke (1995) indeed showed that after four weeks' treatment only seven patients in the placebo group had not responded to treatment.

Nature of placebo response

Placebo effects have characteristics that are strikingly similar to those of active medication. A dose-effect relationship (Blackwell, Bloomfield and Buncher, 1972), time effect curves, cumulated effects after repeated administration and carry-over effects after cessation of placebo administration have been described (Lasagna, Laties and Dohan, 1958). Placebos can also have complex interactions with other (active) medication (Kleijnen *et al.*, 1994).

As pointed out above, placebos can lead to side-effects. They can also produce worsening of symptoms (Shapiro, Wilensky and Struening, 1968) and cases of placebo dependence have been described (Vinar, 1969; Boleloucky, 1971).

Placebos in clinical practice

There are many situations in which placebo use in clinical practice is less harmful and more beneficial than active (drug) treatment (Editorial, 1970). The majority of health care professionals do, in fact, have experience with placebo treatment (Gray and Flynn, 1981). Yet the deliberate use of placebo is an uncomfortable subject that is rarely discussed openly (Wall, 1992). Using placebos outside of clinical trials hints at charlatanism and, perhaps more importantly, it usually involves deceiving the patient. Many physicians therefore feel that deliberate placebo administration is unethical.

But even if one is opposed to prescribing a dummy pill in clinical practice, one might be well advised to maximize the placebo effect that is associated with specific therapy. Whenever we treat patients, the placebo effect is part of the therapeutic response. Depending on the particular situation, one can optimize the placebo response by emphasizing and using one or more of its determinants during the therapeutic encounter. For instance, empathic reassurance will produce better results than truth and uncertainty (Thomas, 1987).

My prediction is that medicine will slowly re-discover the power of the placebo effect and apply it more widely. In order to achieve this aim we must learn to understand the complex phenomena involved and therefore direct rigorous research towards their investigation.

References

Beecher, H.K. (1955) The poweraful placebo. *JAMA*, **159**, 1602–6.

Benedetti, F. (1996) The opposite effects of the opiate antagonist naloxone and the acholecystokinin antagonist proglumide on placebo analgesia. *Pain*, **64**, 535–43.

Blackwell, B., Bloomfield, S.S. and Buncher, C.R. (1972) Demonstration to medical students of placebo responses and non-drug factors. *Lancet*, **1**, 1279–82.

Boleloucky, Z. (1971) A contribution to the problems of placebo dependence: a case report. *Act. Nerv. Super.*, **13**, 190–91.

Bouchet, C., Guillemin, C. and Briacon, S. (1996) Non-specific effects in longitudinal studies. Impact on quality of life measurements. *J. Clin. Epidemiol.*, **49**, 15–20.

Carne, S. (1961) The action of chorionic gonadotrophin in the obese. *Lancet*, **ii**, 1282–4.

Cobb, L.A., Thomas, G.I., Dillard, D.H. *et al.* (1959) An evaluation of internal mammary artery ligation by a double blind technique. *N. Engl. J. Med.*, **260**, 1115–18.

Cromie, B.W. (1963) The feet of clay of the double blind trial. *Lancet*, **9**, 994–7.

Davidson, J. (1996) Self-healing and the placebo response. *Br. Homoeop.*, **85**, 161–2.

Dimond, E.G., Kittle, C.F. and Cockett, J.E. (1960) Comparison of internal mammary artery ligation and sham operation for angina pectoris. *Am. J. Cardiol.*, **4**, 483–6.

Editorial (1970) Placebo effect. *BMJ*, **11**, 437.

Ernst, E. (1992) Placebo forte. *Wien. Med. Wschr.*, **142**, 217–19.

Ernst, E. (1996) Make believe medicine. The amazing powers of placebo. *Eur. J. Phys. Med. Rehab.*, **6(4),** 124–5.
Ernst, E. and Abbot, N.C. (in press). Placebos in clinical practice, results of a survey of nurses.
Ernst, E. and Resch, K.L. (1995a) The concept of the perceived and true placebo effect. *BMJ,* **311**, 551–3.
Ernst, E. and Resch, K.L. (1995b) The importance of placebo effects. *JAMA*, **273**, 283.
Freedman, P. (1995) The clinical trial. *JAMA*, **274**, 51–7.
Fulder, S.J. and Munro, R.E. (1985) Complementary medicine in the United Kingdom: Patients, practitioners and consultations. *Lancet*, 542–5.
Goodwin, J.S., Goodwin, J.M. and Voger, A.V. (1979) Knowledge and use of placebo by house officers and nurses. *Ann. Intern. Med.*, **91**, 106–10.
Gotzsche, P. (1994) Is there logic in the placebo? *Lancet*, **344**, 925–6.
Gracely, R.H., Dubner, R., Deeter, W.R. *et al.* (1985) Clinicians' expectations influence placebo analgesia. *Lancet*, **1**, 43.
Gray, G. and Flynn, P. (1981) A survey of placebo use in general hospital. *Gen. Hosp. Psych.*, **3**, 199–203.
Grenfell, R., Briggs, A.H. and Holland, W.C. (1961) A double-blind study of the treatment of hypertension. *JAMA,* **176**, 124–67.
Grünbaum, A. (1986) The placebo concept in medicine and psychiatry. *Psychol. Med.,* **16**, 19–38.
Hashish, I., Feinman, C. and Harvey, W. (1988) Reduction of postoperative pain and swelling by ultrasound: a placebo effect. *Pain*, **83**, 303–11.
Kaplan, S.H., Greenfield, S. and Ware, J.E. (1989) Assessing the effects of physician–patient interactions on the outcomes of chronic disease. *Med. Care*, **27** (suppl), S110–27.
Kienle, G.S. (1995) *Der sogenannte Placeboeffekt. Illusion, Fakten, Realität.* Stuttgart: Schattaner.
Kirsch, I. (1986) Unsuccessful redefinitions of the term placebo. *Am. Psychol.*, **41**, 844–5.
Kleijnen, J., de Craen, A.J.M., van Everdingen, J. *et al.* (1994) Placebo effect in double-blind clinical trials: a review of interactions with medications. *Lancet*, **344**, 1347–9.
Langley, G.B. and Sheppeard, H. (1987) Transcutaneous electrical nerve stimulation (TNS) and its relationship to placebo therapy: a review. *NZ. Med. J.*, **100**, 215–17.
Lasagna, L., Laties, V.G. and Dohan, J.L. (1958) Further studies on the 'pharmacology' of placebo administration. *J. Clin. Invest.*, **37**, 533–7.
Lepaisart, (1995) Further studies on placebo. *Rev. Franc. Gynecol. Obstet.*, **90**, 94–8.
Lesse, S. (1962) Placebo reactions in psychotherapy. *Dis. Nerv. Syst.*, **12**, 313–19.
Liberman, R. (1961) Analysis of the placebo phenomenon. *J. Chron. Dis.,* **15**, 761–83.
Liberman, R. (1964) An experimental study of the placebo response under three different situations of pain. *J. Psychiat. Res.*, **2**, 233–46.
Luparello, T., Leist, N., Lourie, C.H. *et al.* (1970) The interaction of psychologic stimuli and pharmacologic agents on airway reactivity in asthmatic subjects. *Psychosom. Med.*, **32**, 509–13.
Melchart, D. (1996) Die Plazebo-Verwirrung. *Forsch. Komplementärmed.*, **3**, 109.
Oh, V.M. (1994) The placebo effect: can we use it better? *BMJ,* **309**, 69–70.
Omer, H. and London, P. (1989) Signal and noise in psychotherapy: the role and control of nonspecific factors. *Br. J. Psychiatry*, **155**, 239–45.
Richardson, P.H. (1989) Placebos: their effectiveness and modes of action. In *Health psychology: processes and applications* (A. Broome, ed.), pp. 35–56, London: Chapman and Hall.
Richardson, P.H. (1994) Placebo effects in pain management. *Pain Reviews*, **1**, 15–32.
Rosenzweig, P., Brochier, S. and Zipfel, A. (1993) The placebo effect in healthy volunteers: influence of experimental conditions on the adverse events profile during phase 1 studies. *Clin. Pharmacol. Ther.*, **54**, 578–83.
Ross, M. and Olson, J.M. (1982) Placebo effects in medical research and practice. In *Social Psychology and Behavioural Medicine* (J.R. Eiser, ed.), pp. 441–58, Chichester: Wiley.
Rothman, K. (1996) Placebo mania. *BMJ,* **313**, 3–4.

Saradeth, T., Resch, K.L. and Ernst, E. (1994) Placebo for varicose veins – don't eat it, rub it! *Phlebology*, **9**, 63–6.

Schwitzgebel, R. and Traugott, M. (1968) Initial note on the placebo effect of machines. *Behav. Med.*, **13**, 267–73.

Shapiro, A.K. (1964) Etiological factors in placebo effect. *JAMA*, **187**, 712–14.

Shapiro, A.K. and Morris, L.A. (1978) The placebo effect in medical and psychological therapies. In *Handbook of Psychotherapy and Behavioral Change* (A.E. Bergin and S. Garfield, eds.), pp. 369–410, New York: John Wiley.

Shapiro, A.P., Myers, T., Reiser, M.F. *et al.* (1954) Comparison of blood pressure response to Veriloid and to the doctor. *Psychosom. Med.*, **16**, 478–88.

Shapiro, A.K., Wilensky, H. and Struening, E.L. (1968) Study of the placebo effect with a placebo test. *Compr. Psychiatry*, **9**, 118–37.

Sternbach, R.A. (1964) The effects of instructional sets on autonomic responsivity. *Psychophysiology*, **1**, 67–72.

Tangrea, J.A., Adrianza, E. and Helsel, W.E. (1994) Risk factors for the development of placebo adverse reactions in a multicenter clinical trial. *Ann. Epidemiol.*, **4**, 327–31.

Taub, H.A., Mitchell, J.N., Stuber, F.E., Eisenberg, L., Beard, M.C. and McCormack, R.K. (1979) Analgesia for operative dentistry: A comparison of acupuncture and placebo. *Oral Surg.*, **48(3)**, 205–10.

Thomas, K.B. (1987) General practice consultations: is there any point in being positive? *BMJ*, **294**, 1200–02.

Turner, J.A., Deyo, R.A., Loeser, J.D. *et al.* (1994) The importance of placebo effects in pain treatment and research. *JAMA*, **271**, 1609–14.

Uhlenhuth, E.H., Canter, A., Neustadt, J.O. *et al.* (1959) The symptomatic relief of anxiety with meprobamate, phenobarbital and placebo. *Am. J. Psychiatry*, **115**, 905–10.

Vinar, O. (1969) Dependence on a placebo: a case report. *Br. J. Psychiatry*, **115**, 1189–90.

Wall, P.D. (1992) The placebo effect, an unpopular topic. *Pain*, **51**, 1–3.

Wickramasekera, I. (1977) The placebo effect and medical instruments and biofeedback. *J. Clin. Eng.*, **2**, 227–30.

Wiesenauer, M. and Lüdtke, R. (1995) The treatment of pollinosis with Galphimia galauca D4. *Phytomed.*, **2**, 3–6.

Chapter 8

Is homoeopathy a placebo response? What if it is? What if it is not?

David Reilly

Introduction

The question 'Is homoeopathy a placebo response?' generates two hypotheses:

It is (*solely* a placebo response).
It is not (solely a placebo response).

All might agree homoeopathy must in part be a placebo (because all care is), but is it also more? This in turn mainly comes down to asking, do homoeopathic drugs when diluted beyond Avogadro's point show biological activity?

What evidence is available for the 'It is' and the 'It is not' hypotheses?

There is now sufficient circumstantial weight for both hypotheses, so both require experimental verification – neither can be given a 'special case' status of 'intuitive' obviousness; proof is required. Some proof exists for both hypotheses.

What are the implications for homoeopathy?

The central issue is that there are major implications to be faced *which ever* hypothesis is correct. Is homoeopathy an effective, non-toxic, acceptable therapy being ignored and under-exploited? Or is it a well developed system for producing 'placebo' responses – that is intention modified self healing responses (IMoHRs).

Medical care must now consider the implication that enhanced human healing, with less side effects, can be achieved with better time and therapeutic consultations. In addition, if the homoeopathic dilutions are proven active, an additional dimension to therapy and science opens up; and if the dilutions are purely placebos, the implications for research which must be faced is that the placebo controlled clinical trial process is producing alarming rates of false positive results.

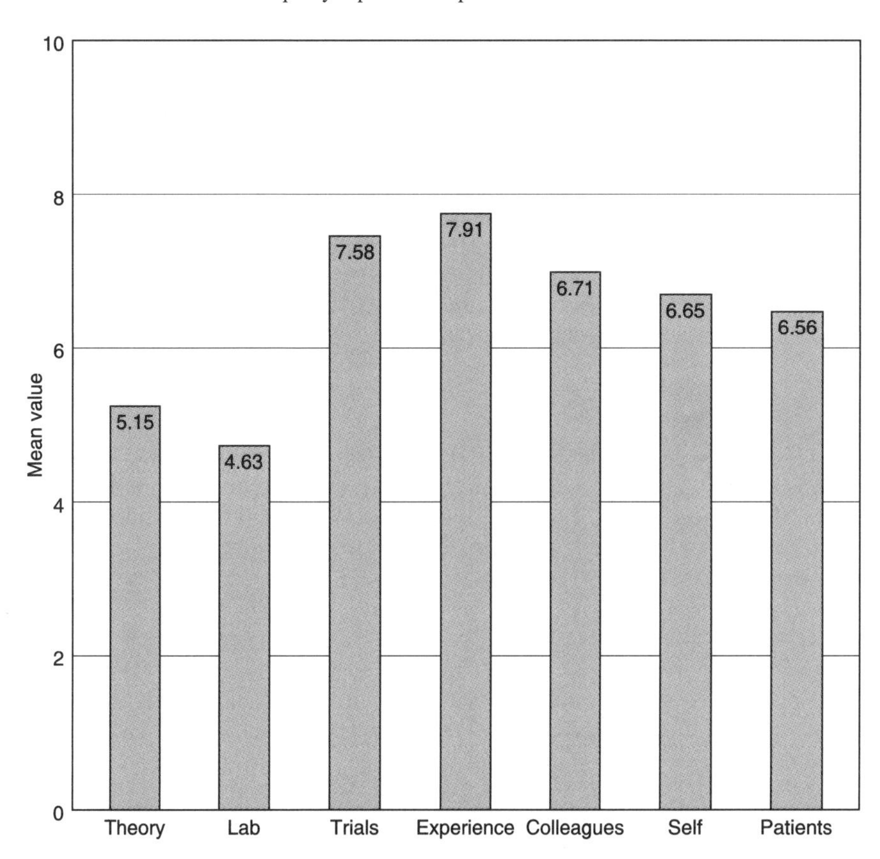

Figure 8.1 Validating complementary medicine. What sort of evidence? Views of 210 trainee GPs at the XI National GP Trainee Conference, July 1987 when asked 'What sort of validation or evidence do you consider important before you would accept an alternative technique as useful for your patients?'

The challenges, the questions and the two hypotheses

Homoeopathy works; that is, patients and carers at times benefit from it. Why?

Although this statement and the resultant question are disarmingly simple, these clinical phenomena and the question asked of them are not. Human care can be very tough to understand, and evidence is often complex and multi-dimensional, a mosaic. There is an increasing recognition of this complexity, and Figure 8.1 offers an example of an 'evidence profile' (Reilly and Taylor, 1993, pp. 11–12) demanded by a group of doctors when asked what sort of proof they wanted before they would use a complementary and alternative medicine (CAM) therapy in their patients. As you can see from the results, in their proof empiricism dominates over theory, interlaced with others forms of evidence, with no avenue discounted. In practice different audiences can require different evidence profiles for a given subject, determined by who is making the enquiry, and why.

At this time in history the primary question evoked by a scientific audience when presented with homoeopathy's claims usually boils down to asking, 'Do homoeopathic drugs when diluted beyond Avogadro's point show biological activity?' Yet their voice is only one in this enquiry. Beyond their primary question lies a myriad of puzzles and challenges, some of which will be of even greater interest to other audiences, who may hold different attitudes towards evidence – perhaps health purchasers interested in cost issues, legislators concerned about safety, or carers wondering why homoeopathic consultations are so effective.

The two hypotheses

Yet around this central debate lie core issues of interest to everyone involved in health care – and the contention of this chapter is that it is time to grasp the nettle of these issues. The title I have used is intended to focus our minds by reframing the primary question 'Is homoeopathy a placebo response?' into the two hypotheses it generates:

1. Homoeopathy is solely placebo, or
2. It is not.

I put it this stark way to make it clear that which ever hypothesis is correct it carries profound implications for medicine and science that should not be ignored.

The evidence for each of the two hypotheses needs weighed (and much of it is covered elsewhere in this book), and the implication of each conclusion considered in its own light.

The evidence for the two hypotheses

There is now sufficient circumstantial weight for both hypotheses, so both require experimental verification – neither can be given a 'special case' status of 'intuitive' obviousness. While all might agree homoeopathy must be in part a placebo (because all care is), the issue is, is it also more?

Table 8.1 sketches some of the forms of evidence available which might assist you in organizing your enquiry. Here I will just comment on a few aspects of the points in the table.

Theoretical evidence

Theoretically a case can be made for each link in the chain of the homoeopathic process. An accepted everyday example of the central issue of counter-stimulant therapy would be pollen therapy in hay fever (a branch of the homoeopathic approach), and here hormetic effects (Stebbing, 1982) offers a model for this. For understanding the claim of powerful whole-organism effects being triggered by receiving and amplifying amazingly tiny quantities of qualitative stimuli, nature offers the model of pheromones

Table 8.1 Is homoeopathy a placebo response? What if it is? What if it is not? The evidence

	If it *is* solely a placebo response	*Is*	*Is not*	If it is *not* solely a placebo response
Theory				
A priori plausibility	'Inherently unlikely'	++++	+	A case can be made
Biochemical	Beyond Avogadro's	++++	0	No chance
Biophysical	Not obvious	++	++	Some theories
Theory of science	Caution in order	0	0	'If?' before 'How?'
Practice				
Historical use	Could be placebo	++	+	Circumstantial
Current use	Fashion, naivete	++	++	Suggestive
Animal use	Placebo effects might occur	+	++	Less placebo response than humans
Clinic	Unclear	+	++	Challenging, useful results, but why?
Experimental				
Placebo research	All the phenomenon of healing, and therefore homoeopathy, can be provoked or modified by placebo	++++	++++	Homoeopathy may catalyse and enhance the same mechanisms as placebo (see Trials)
Laboratory research	Only unreliable, poorly reproducible results	++	++	2:1 positive to negative results
Controlled trials	Critical mass of evidence needed? Publication bias reducing as likely explanation of balance of positive results	+	+++	Critical mass of evidence needed? 150 or so RCTs to date, about 3:1 in favour of a 'more than placebo' action. (Daily care will need more and different evidence.)

Table 8.2

Audit of 100 out patients in Glasgow Homoeopathic Hospital
100 sequential patients from July 1992
Followed up after 1 year with 80% returns

At presentation:
81% had failed to respond to conventional treatment
47% had seen a consultant for the problem

After 1 year:
60% improved in the presenting complaint
61% improved in well being
49% had a sustained improvement of value in daily living
37% had a sustained reduction in conventional therapy.

Audit of 100 in patients at Glasgow Homoeopathic Hospital

At presentation:
100% had already had conventional care
97% had seen a consultant for the problem
67% had previously needed to be hospitalized for the problem

At a mean of 3 months after treatment (with a 73% response rate):
58% had a useful improvement in the presenting complaint
67% had a useful improvement in general mood and well being.

(air-borne informational molecules). However, in terms of the high dilutions of homoeopathy, they are evidently nonsense from a biochemical perspective – but they make some sense if thought of as biophysical informational patterning, like the recording of a computer file on magnetic tape without a change in chemical composition, or the wonderful individuality of snowflakes which do not differ chemically from their neighbours.

But however interesting these ideas are, they cannot prove or disprove empirical (and unexplained) fact.

Evidence from practice

The second section of Table 8.1 touches on the evidence from clinical practice. The historic persistence of clinical effects raises as many questions as it answers, but to help put it in a contemporary context Table 8.2 restates the puzzle by showing the useful clinical outcomes that patients report one year after attending expert homoeopathic clinics. The majority of patients said there was a persistent response of value in daily living – and yet this was when most had resorted to homoeopathy after the benefits of conventional care had plateaued.

To further emphasize the fundamental nature of the challenge from clinical practice Figure 8.2 shows a graph of the reported value of a homoeopathic treatment used by conventional primary care workers after receiving simple foundation level training in Glasgow (Reilly *et al.*, 1995).

About 20 per cent of Scotland's general practitioners have completed basic homoeopathic training and they are reporting continued use and benefit from integrating this therapy with conventional practice. This benefit is reported as covering both clinical results, and the quality of care and consultations (Reilly and Taylor, 1993, pp. 29–31; Reilly, 1995).

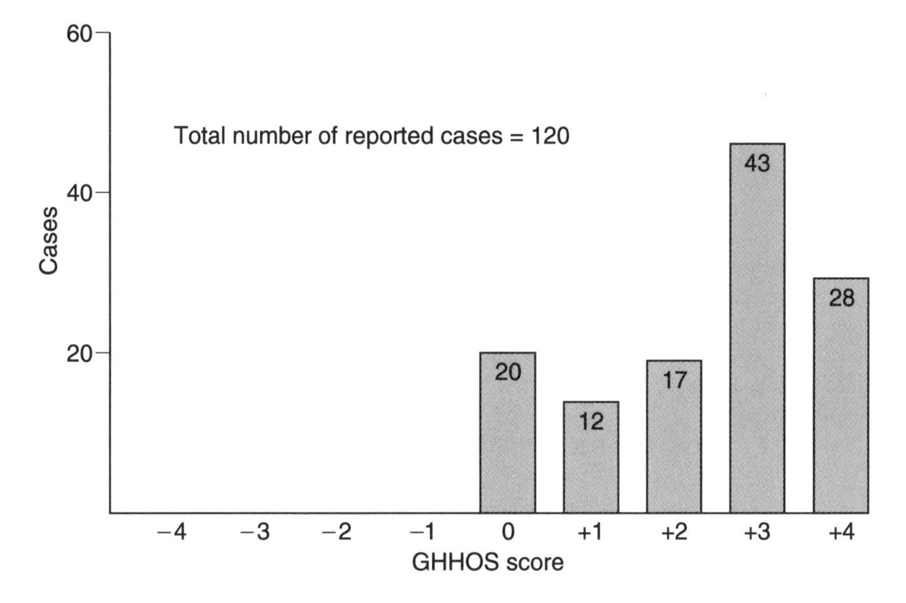

Provisional outcome measure of 73% ≥ +2

Glasgow Homoeopathic Hospital outcome and satisfaction scales

GHH outcome scale		GHH patient satisfaction scale
Cured/back to normal	+4	Complete satisfaction
Major improvement	+3	Major satisfaction
Moderate improvement, affecting daily living	+2	Moderate satisfaction
Slight improvement, no effect on daily living	+1	Slight satisfaction
No change/unsure	0	No satisfaction
Slight deterioration, no effect on daily living	−1	Slight dissatisfaction
Moderate deterioration, affecting daily living	−2	Moderate dissatisfaction
Major deterioration	−3	Major dissatisfaction
Disastrous deterioration	−4	Complete dissatisfaction

Figure 8.2 Analysis of the early returns of the data collection project using the GHHOS to measure outcome. The use of ARNICA in trauma and injury.

Experimental evidence

Table 8.1 goes on to sketch the issues of the experimental evidence for these theoretical and practical phenomena.

Placebo evidence: IMoHR

There is no doubt in my mind that all of the healing phenomena of homoeopathy can be induced by placebo alone, but the question is complex because homoeopathy may stimulate the very same mechanisms as placebo, giving a synergistic effect. Before proceeding I would like to suggest that placebo should be re-considered, and if necessary re-named, to recognize that the term is being used to cover an orchestra of healing responses modified by the intention and circumstances of the healing encounter. For now I will call this an intention modified self healing response (IMoHR) effect, and would say that this might be the sole catalyst of change in a care event, or it might be interactive with the specific therapy effect (i.e. Therapy + IMoHR = TIMoHR).

Figure 8.3 gives evidence from an asthma trial conducted at Glasgow University for my statement that placebo (IMoHR) effects can reproduce the phenomena of homoeopathy (Reilly and Taylor, 1993). As you can see patients produced aggravations and ameliorations from placebo along with the homoeopathic phenomena of direction of cure and return of old symptoms being provoked. Opposite actions from two identical placebos in the same patient were noted, perhaps mediated by a change in the clinician's expectation of outcome at the point of the double-blind prescription.

I would contend that these phenomena are intrinsic to healing – irrespective of how mobilized – be it spontaneously or triggered, and irrespective of the triggers – be they specific or non-specific. Our focus should be as much on the healing as on the trigger.

More-than-placebo evidence: TIMoHR

But what evidence is there that homoeopathy is greater than placebo alone – that it is a TIMoHR, not IMoHR effect? Here we turn to the evidence from placebo controlled trials and the meta-analyses of them (Kleijnen, Knipschild and ter Riet, 1991). As summarized in Figure 8.4, the Glasgow team's experiences echo those of other workers around the world: the randomized placebo controlled trial is tending to come out in favour of homoeopathy (Reilly *et al.*, 1994). We have discovered in a series of placebo controlled trial and resulting meta-analysis, that we have produced positive results – with predictability and reproducibility – which appear to confirm homoeopathic action over and above its placebo effect. We have failed to find the evidence we sought for the counter 'placebo only' hypothesis.

To date the laboratory evidence is uncertain but meta-analyses are again tending to favour the idea of a biological action to form the dilutions (Linde *et al.*, 1994). This evidence is considered elsewhere in this book.

The implications of the two hypotheses

We now turn to the implications of the two hypotheses and the evidence. This is the most challenging area. Some of the implications are outlined in Table 8.3.

Implications of the first hypothesis: if homoeopathy is solely placebo

If the first hypothesis is proven correct and homoeopathy is solely a placebo response we would have to consider that good clinical results can be obtained

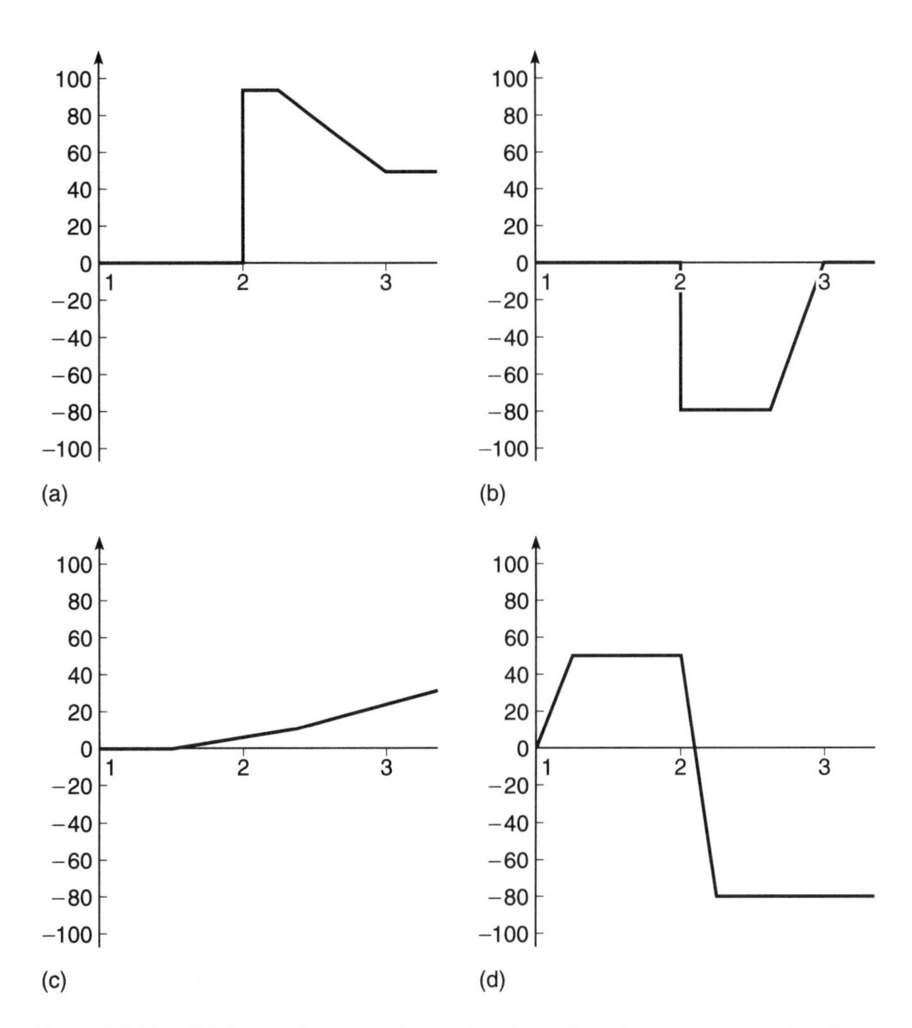

Figure 8.3 The OPIC: overall progress interactive chart. Overall progress interactive charts completed interactively by patient and doctor at each monthly visit, so that by the end of the study they had charted the severity of asthma over 12 weeks. On a scale of ± 100% a rise is an improvement and the line descends in a deterioration. The first point on the horizontal axis marks the prescription of a single-blind placebo. Four weeks on at point 2 the patient has been given, randomized and double blind, either a second placebo or active homoeopathy. At point 3 a third prescription is given only if required; of course those randomized to the placebo group would again receive a placebo treatment. (a) No response to the first single-blind placebo. Dramatic improvement within hours to the double-blind randomized prescription – ran a marathon! Waned to 50% within about a month. (b) No response to the first single-blind placebo. Dramatic aggravation within hours to the double-blind randomized prescription. 'Worst ever', plus return of old symptoms (rhinitis) and a new symptom of mid-thoracic back pain. (c) No response to the first single-blind placebo. A smooth and sustained improvement to the double-blind randomized prescription. (d) Marked improvement with the first single-blind placebo. Dramatic aggravation within hours to the double-blind randomized prescription. Only patient (c) received active medicine at point 2. All other prescriptions were placebos.

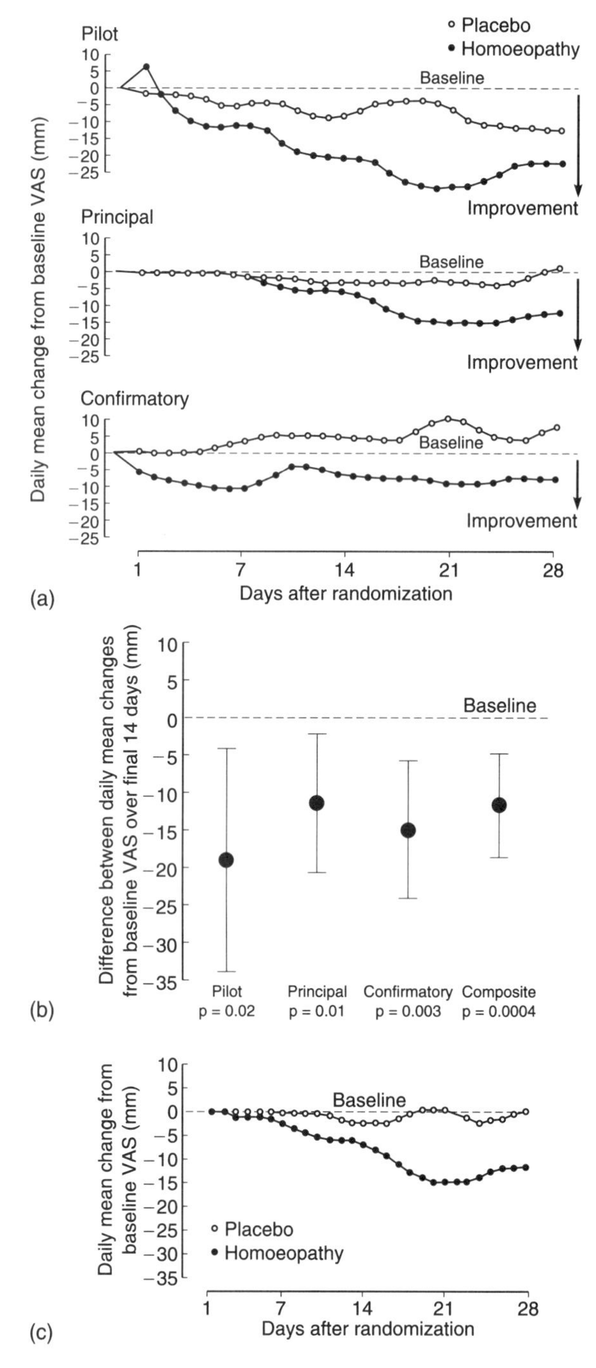

Figure 8.4 Figures taken from Reilly *et al.* 1994. The trials (pilot and principle in hay fever, confirmatory in asthma) used homoeopathic allergen desensitization as a model to test the placebo hypothesis and the reproducibility of the evidence in favour of homoeopathy. (a) Pattern of change within each trial. (b) Trials compared and combined. 95% CI and difference between means. (c) Composite of the three trials.

Table 8.3 Is homoeopathy a placebo response? What if it is? What if it is not? The implications

	If it *is* solely a placebo response	*Is*	*Is not*	If it is *not* solely a placebo response
THE DILUTIONS				
Basic sciences, e.g. bio/physics, bio/chemistry	No problem	0	+ + +	Major expansion of understanding
Randomized, double-blind, placebo controlled trials	?Discredited – predictable, reproducible false positives	+ + + +	+ +	Vindicated as a useful empirical tool
Future science	Lessons in folly	+ +	+ + + +	Imaging, measuring, understanding the effects – new developments
THE CARE				
Our understanding				
Mind-body medicine, psychoneuroimmunology 'placebo': intention modified healing responses (IMoHR)	200 years of studying this.	+ + + +	+ +	Insight into whole-person care, disease and healing
Our practice				
Results	Problem for patients and carers; what will survive without the ritual? (see Side effects)	+ + +	+ + + +	New ways of care
Time with carer	Time heals	+ + +	+ + + +	More time needed
Side effects	Many orthodox drugs are being used when placebos would suffice; seek other simpler treatments	+ + +	+ + + +	A safer alternative to often be used first line with current drugs more now second line
Patients				
Self healing	Encourage awareness	+ + + +	+ + + +	Encourage awareness
Satisfaction	Confused	+ + + +	+ + + +	Enhanced
Purchasers	Problem – what to substitute?	+ + + +	+ + + +	Useful, safer additional option – ?cost impact

at less cost and side effects than those of orthodox care by placebo/IMoHR effects through time and effective consultations.

- Is conventional medicine ready to take the daunting implications of this on board? If we are producing poorer results and more side effects by the way we approach our patients and our systems of care, will we reform them and the educational and administrative structures which support them? Will we take on board the whole person and mind-body perspective this change would call for? Will we give more time and put in more effort to produce therapeutic relationships?
- Would homoeopathic practitioners and patients face the implications of the power of healing encounters? This will be especially difficult for those who currently tend to over invest in the prescription as the agent of change, disregarding the other rich healing elements which homoeopathy can bring.
- What of science? We would need to conclude that the placebo controlled trial process is showing discrediting rates of false positives. About 70 per cent of studies would have been showing false positives in what would then be understood to actually have been trials of one placebo against another (Anon, 1994). Can researchers produce the results they want despite double blinding, and if so, how? What would then need to be done to change conventional treatment assessment?

Implications of the second hypothesis: homoeopathy is shown to have a greater than placebo action

Compared to the implications of Hypothesis 1, in some ways this is the simpler scenario:

- Scientific vision and theory would need to expand to embrace informational carriage by liquids.
- Medicine would have a whole range of new therapeutic tools available to integrate with the other healing arts. These would be safer than current drugs and when appropriate could be used first line, reserving biochemical therapies as second line.
- For future care and research, avenues would be opened up of interventions as subtle and powerful as nature, with lasting, transforming impact on biological responses from fine and subtle signals far nearer to nature's own than our current drugs.
- There would be an encouragement of whole person (and animal) perspectives in care and practical applications of the newly emerging psychoneuroimmune understanding: a field which homoeopathy has explored in a practical way for 200 years.

Implications of both hypotheses

The implications are exciting and challenging whatever way we look at them for both the art and science of medicine. There is an enormous amount to learn and develop from this vision and system of care which respects and works with therapeutic encounters and the subtlety of healing. And if the dilutions are proven active, even more amazing perspectives will unfold.

References

Anon. (1994) Reilly's challenge. (Editorial) *Lancet*, **344**, 1585.

Kleijnen, J., Knipschild, P. and ter Riet, G. (1991) Clinical trials of Homoeopathy. *Br. Med. J.*, **302**, 316–23.

Linde, K., Jonas, W.B., Worke, D.M.F., Wagner, H. and Eifel, F. (1994) Critical review and meta-analysis of serial agitated dilutions in experimental toxicology. *Human and Experimental Toxicology*, **13**, 481–92.

Reilly, D.T. (1995) Clarifying competence by defining its limits. Lessons from the Glasgow Educational Model of Homoeopathic Training. *Complementary Therapies in Medicine*, **3**, 21–4.

Reilly, D., Duncan, R.S, Leckridge, R. *et al.* (1995) IDCCIM – International Data Collection Centres for Integrative Medicine. University of Exeter 2nd Annual Symposium on Complementary Health Care. December 1995.

Reilly, D.T. and Taylor, M.A. (1993) Developing Integrated Medicine. Report of the RCCM Research Fellowship in Complementary Medicine, Glasgow University 1987–90. *Complementary Therapies in Medicine*, **1**, Suppl. 1, 1–49.

Reilly, D.T., Taylor, M.A., Campbell, J., Beattie, N., McSharry, C., Aitchison, T., Carter, R. and Stevenson, R. (1994) Is evidence for homoeopathy reproducible? *Lancet*, **344**, 1601–6.

Stebbing, A.R.D. (1982) Hormesis – The stimulation of growth by low levels of inhibitors. *The Science of the Total Environment*, **22**, 213–34.

Chapter 9

Safety in homoeopathy

Wayne B. Jonas

Introduction

Homoeopathy involves the application of extremely small doses of substances diluted in a serial fashion and succussed or agitated between dilutions. These preparations are selected by producing drug pictures or images through the administration of medications to healthy individuals and matching and applying these to those with similar symptoms who are ill.

Originally, the founder of homoeopathy, Samuel Hahnemann (1755 to 1843), began diluting his drugs in order to reduce toxic side effects. He and others claimed that when such drugs were carefully matched to the patients, the serial-agitated dilutions lost their toxic effects, yet still retained stimulatory therapeutic effects. It was subsequently discovered that many homoeopathic preparations no longer have the possibility of any original molecules left in them. The conventional reaction to this is that they can have no specific effects at all; that is, they are all placebo, either therapeutic or toxic, and therefore are at least harmless. This attitude is reflected in the approach taken by the Food and Drug Administration of the United States, that generally classifies homoeopathic preparations as over-the-counter drugs approved for sale without claims of effectiveness, and exempt from the standard toxicity and safety testing required of other medications.

Recent evidence indicates that homoeopathic medications may not work in identical fashion to placebo. If these claims are substantiated and homoeopathic remedies are felt to produce specific effects, then the possibility exists that they also may produce specific adverse effects. In this regard, their evaluation will require the same assessment of risk benefit ratio as any other intervention. A review of the conceptual issues in the safety of complementary medicine has previously been done (Jonas, 1997). General safety issues can be classified as direct, indirect, involving misclassification and paradigmatic or interpretation issues. These classifications also provide a useful framework for assessing safety issues in homoeopathy.

Safety assessment

Unfortunately, the current state-of-the-art in safety screening, even in conventional medicine, is far from satisfactory. Clinical studies are generally set up to assess drug effectiveness identified through pre-selected outcome measures using control groups to test specific hypotheses. Adverse or so-called side effects are collected on the side, as it were, and are subject to the multiple errors and biases that afflict any unsystematic and uncontrolled means of data collection. For example:

1 Because so-called side effects are often not pre-defined, there is a risk of data dredging from multiple outcomes collection.
2 Because safety issues are generally restricted to small numbers of patients, the risk exists of identifying chance effects and missing other effects.
3 Because most studies are of short duration, more global, long-term effects on overall health are usually not assessed.
4 Rare and idiosyncratic effects that occur after prolonged use or in only one out of less than every few thousand patients will usually not be detected.

Thus, the current state-of-the-art in adverse-effect reporting is often limited to implication by analogy from laboratory and animal studies, case reports and case series supplemented with occasional post-marketing surveillance, without pre-determined outcome measurements. The situation in the assessment of safety in homoeopathy is even worse as even these minimal approaches are usually not found.

Direct safety

Direct safety effects usually refer to direct toxic effects from a drug itself or adverse reactive effects to a drug. Many of the homoeopathic drug pictures are produced by a process called 'proving' in which homoeopathic preparations are given to healthy individuals and the symptoms produced are recorded. This is analogous to a Phase 1 trial and demonstrates an assumed direct adverse effect from stimulation by homoeopathic remedies. Very little animal research is done to test whether such adverse effects occur in a more objective way. However, when this has been done, it has not indicated an innocuous nature even of very high dilutions. For example:

- Stearnes (1928) examined the effects of very high dilutions of *naturum muriticum* on several generations of guinea pigs. He showed that compared to a control group, guinea pigs given repeated daily doses of high dilutions of *naturum muriticum* became unhealthy, lost their hair, were less alert, lost weight, and began to stop breeding.
- Dwarakanath (1979) reported a study in which the homoeopathic remedy China, in the 200C and 1000C potency, produced acute reductions in body temperature measured rectally in rats compared to a control group.
- Prasa and Chandrasekhar (1980) reported that high potencies of *Pulsatilla* M and 10M administered immediately before and after mating induced lymphocytic infiltration of the implanted fetus and fetal reabsorption compared to controls.
- Kumar and co-workers (1981) reported that high potencies of *Caulophytum* retarded uterine ovarian cell maturation and stimulated endometrial proliferation. Similar results have been reported in other animal experiments.

Although these research studies are few and often of low quality, they indicate that one cannot assume high potencies of homoeopathic remedies have no direct toxic effects. This brings into question the minimum toxic dose approach to screening for safety of homoeopathy in which the perceived minimum toxic dose in a potency is assumed to be safe under all conditions.

Reactive adverse effects are also reported in homoeopathy. It is commonly claimed that 'aggravations' or enhancement of symptoms occurs after selection of the right remedy. These, of course, are adverse effects. Unfortunately, the frequency of aggravations has not been systematically studied.

Reilly, in a systematic study of high dilutions of allergens showed that approximately 24 per cent of patients reported such aggravations (Reilly *et al.*, 1986). This resulted in about a 6 per cent drop-out rate from the study due to such adverse effects. Sensitive patients are said to often produce severe aggravations. The author has seen a case of sudden severe aggravation of asthma necessitating hospitalization from homoeopathic treatment.

Finally, reactive adverse effects include a variety of idiosyncratic effects, such as allergies, and other kinds of effects that may not occur except very rarely or after long periods of time.

Indirect effects

The second category of adverse effects are those of indirect effects. The bulk of these effects probably occur from false negative results and neglect. If an effective therapy exists, then treatment with ineffective therapy, be it homoeopathy or otherwise, will result in unnecessary progression of the disease and adverse effects. Simply demonstrating that a drug works differently from placebo is insufficient to assess adverse effect. A drug response over one placebo may not be the same as another drug over another placebo. Only direct comparisons of two interventions can give us information on optimal therapies, and thus the degree of neglect effects that occur through the administration of sub-optimal therapies. Some homoeopaths claim there is a duration of action from particular potencies, even up to a year after a single dose. The author has seen cases in which individuals with chronic illness, such as gingivitis and gall bladder disease, have been told to wait for the full duration of action of the remedy, resulting in continued suffering. Homoeopaths also claim that the return of symptoms are often a good sign, but for most individuals this is not desirable. This would also be classified as an indirect effect.

Symptom control without resolution is another indirect effect. Again, the only evidence for this comes from case reports. For example:

- A woman with post-operative staples left in the skin was treating the pain with the homoeopathic remedy *hypericum*. This resulted in the staples being left in and undiscovered for longer than would have happened without pain control.
- A woman was effectively treating what she thought were menstrual cramps, with a homoeopathic remedy. It was later discovered that she had a ruptured ovarian cyst and was bleeding internally.

Such effects, of course, can occur with any kind of misdiagnosis and probably occur more often with conventional medicine.

There are certain conditions which require immediate attention and which modern medicine clearly has ways of managing, such as acute myocardial infarction, fractures and bacterial meningitis. The attempt to use homoeopathic medications in these conditions will in most cases result in adverse outcomes.

Likewise, the lack of use of effective homoeopathic medications when available will result in undue suffering. Failure to use arnica, for example, in cases of trauma may be such an example, although there are currently insufficient trials to definitively recommend such therapy. The use of homoeopathy in acceleration of the resolution of post-operative ileus, however, has been demonstrated (Dorfman *et al.*, 1992). Failure to use homoeopathy in these situations may result in prolonged post-operative ileus (GRECHO, 1987).

Dose-dependent reverse effects

Dose-dependent reverse effects may also be an example of indirect effects from homoeopathic preparations. Doutremepuich *et al.* (1990) have demonstrated in several models that serially-agitated preparations of aspirin can induce rather than inhibit thrombosis. Animal studies have shown that high potencies of arsenic can accelerate the elimination of arsenic when given in toxic doses (Boiron, 1985; Cazin, Cazin and Boiron, 1987). This brings up the question of whether homoeopathic preparations of essential minerals and nutrients might also stimulate the elimination of such nutrients. If dose-dependent reverse effects occur in a general manner, one needs to ask whether cytotoxic drugs, when given in homoeopathic preparations, might stimulate cellular proliferation and carcinogenesis rather than inhibit it.

Misclassification

Adverse effects can also arise from misclassification, largely due to false positive diagnosis. The classical homoeopathic approach considers the 'totality' of symptoms in the assessment and treatment of a case. One can spend an hour to an hour and a half getting all the patient's symptoms and giving a remedy. Six weeks later, the vast majority of them are likely to have regressed due to spontaneous remission or statistical regression to the mean or other factors. The remedy will appear to have been successful, thus giving a false sense of efficacy. Repeated experiences such as this can result in treatment addiction. The patient returns to have further symptoms assessed and apparently resolved through such non-specific means. This risks degeneration of the therapeutic interaction into worry management. The patient attempts to resolve all symptoms or reduce all risks resulting in repeated visits to the physician. This then is an adverse effect.

A similar phenomenon may occur through the electro-dermal diagnostic techniques that use homoeopathic remedies for treatments. Electrical potential changes on certain points on the fingers and toes of an individual are claimed to be related to early internal health problems. These electro-dermal changes then become diagnostic categories in themselves, requiring treatment with repeated visits and unnecessary medication. This results in the fabrication of illness and may risk the assumption that treatment of these electrical potentials or other outcome measures will prevent health care problems in the future. If patients then neglect well-known lifestyle and other prevention activities, such as exercise, appropriate diet, smoking cessation, etc., they may assume they are at lower risk than they actually are. This may result in potential adverse effects from failure to take steps to prevent illness in the future.

Paradigmatic issues and safety in homoeopathy

Whether a particular effect is classified as beneficial or adverse often depends upon the interpretation of the system and/or the individual involved with that therapy. For example, aggravations in conventional medicine would be classified as adverse, but in homoeopathy are often felt to be a beneficial sign. They indicate an individual's healing processes have been stimulated, and that the person will return to balance and improve in the future.

Homoeopathic literature talks frequently about suppression or symptom shifting in which superficial treatment or symptom control results in deeper and more serious symptoms arising later. Classical homoeopathic literature describes some of the most serious suppression arising from homoeopathic treatment itself in the hands of incompetent practitioners. The assessment and verification of this as an adverse effect is extremely difficult. No systematic data of this appears to be available.

As mentioned, the homoeopathic system often sees the return of old symptoms in a positive light, interpreting it as a good sign rather than as an adverse effect. Patients, however, may not interpret the return of old pains as positive. The more important issue arises about the interpretation of the return of old pathological conditions. For example, a woman treated for a chronic pelvic inflammatory disease had her pain successfully resolved. A vaginal discharge occurred that tested positive for trichomonas. The homoeopath felt it should not be treated topically or specifically as it was a return of an old problem and would resolve with continued homoeopathic treatment. It is completely unknown whether old pathologies might also return in serious conditions, such as cancer, asthma or other diseases.

Finally, the homoeopathic literature also talks of so-called grafting. This is a type of permanent proving in which sensitive individuals given high doses of a remedy have symptoms produced that are prolonged and may be serious. While these are rare according to the homoeopathic literature, such a claim certainly would be classified as an adverse effect.

Conclusion

Safety in homoeopathy cannot be assumed without empirical testing and verification. It involves multiple general categories as in other areas of complementary and conventional medicine. Systematic evaluation of the direct, indirect, misclassification and paradigmatic issues of homoeopathic treatment is necessary. These issues include:

1 the assessment of toxic and reactive direct effects,
2 assessment of the degree and seriousness of false negative diagnoses and neglect,
3 assessment of the degree and rate of false positive diagnoses,
4 failure to use efficacious homoeopathic therapy,
5 clarification of the paradigmatic and interpretation issues around aggravation, suppression, grafting, provings, and returnable symptoms,
6 duration of action of the drug.

Only a systematic approach to evaluating safety in homoeopathy will clarify these issues.

References

Boiron, J. (1985) Comparaison de l'action de Arsenicum album 7 CH normal et chauffé a 120°C sur l'intoxication arsenicale provoquee. *Homéopathie*, **2**, 49–53.

Cazin, J.C., Cazin, M. and Boiron, J. (1987) A study of the effect of decimal and centesimal dilutions of arsenic on the retention of mobilization or arsenic in rats. *Human Toxicology*, **135**(6), 315–20.

Dorfman, P., Amodeo, C., Ricciotti, F., Tetau, M. and Veroux, G. (1992) Illeus post-operatoire et homéopathie: bilan d'une evaluation clinique. *Cahiers de Biotherapie*, **20**, 99–105.

Doutremepuich, C., De Seze, O., Le Roy, D., Lalanne, M.C. and Anne, M.C. (1990) Aspirin at very ultra low dosage in healthy volunteers: effects on bleeding time, platelet aggregation and coagulation. *Haemostasis*, **20**, 99–105.

Dwarakanath, S.K. (1979) Short-term observation on the effects of China in relation to the rectal temperature of albino rats. *Hahnamannian Gleanings*, **6**, 37–41.

GRECHO (1987) Protocole d'un essai de traitement homéopathieque en chirurgie digestive. *La presse medicale*, **16**, 192–3.

Jonas, W.B. (1997) Safety in complementary medicine. In *Complementary Medicine: An Objective Appraisal*, ed. E. Ernst, pp. 126–49. Oxford: Butterworth Heinemann.

Kumar, S., Srivastava, A.K. and Chandrasekhar, K. (1981) The effects of *Caulophytum* on the uterus and ovaries of adult rats. *British Homoeopathic Journal*, **70**, 3, 135–43.

Prasa, S. and Chandrasekhar, K. (1980) Parallel effects of pulsitill and exogenous leutocyclin on the rat ovary, uterus and thyroid, *British Homoeopathic Journal*, **69**, 265–75.

Reilly, D.T., Taylor, M.A., McSharry, C. and Aitchinson, T. (1986) Is homoeopathy a placebo response? Controlled trial of homoeopathic potency, with pollen in hayfever as model. *Lancet*, **ii** (8512), 881–5.

Stearnes, G.B. (1928) Studies in high dilutions. *Homoeopathic Recorder*, **63**, 11, 669–73.

Chapter 10

Reports of complications in homoeopathic treatment

Christian Hentschel, Ralf Kohnen and Eckhart G. Hahn

Introduction

Among the countries of Europe, the popularity of homoeopathy varies considerably. While in Denmark, only about 6 million a year are spent on homoeopathic remedies, the corresponding figure in France is 230 million, and in Germany 210 million (Fischer and Ward, 1994). Both the effectiveness and harmlessness of homoeopathic forms of treatment have still not yet been adequately investigated. The view that the absence of a toxicological risk makes it possible for homoeopathic therapy to induce serious undesired effects can at present neither be affirmed nor negated. Severe adverse reactions have reportedly been observed in association with homoeopathic remedies administered to treat, among other things, dermatological problems. Aberer (1991) published a report on three patients in whom homoeopathic treatment led to very severe skin reactions and, in one patient, even to a need for treatment in an intensive care unit. Aberer was able to reproduce the reactions in these patients by repeating the administration of the homoeopathic remedy. In 1991, Benmeir described a patient with a melanoma who, subsequent to receiving exclusive postoperative treatment with homoeopathic remedies, developed a recurrent tumour weighing 1.8 kg! The primary tumour – which has been excised – had infiltrated to a depth of only 1.74 mm.

Material and method

Within the period between 1 April 1995 and 31 March 1996, all patients attending referred to the emergency room/intensive care unit of Medical Dep. I at the University of Erlangen were questioned about earlier or current treatment with homoeopathic remedies.

These cases were analysed in an attempt to detect possible causal relationships between the homoeopathic treatment and the symptoms that had led to emergency hospitalization.

Results

Within a one year period, a total of 3447 patients (1918 women and 1529 men, average age of 6.4 years) were interviewed. Thirty-nine of these patients died in the emergency room or in the ICU.

The individual cases receiving simultaneous homoeopathic treatment (n = 63; 1.87%) were broken down by indication as shown in Table 10.1.

Despite a thorough diagnostic work-up, including X-rays, ultrasound, etc., no underlying organic pathological findings were detected in 25 of these 63 patients, and the patients themselves attributed their complaints to the homoeopathic treatment they had received.

Of the 25 patients, 18 were women and 7 men. Their average age was 48.90 years (women 49.9, men 46.4 years), and they had received conventional treatment for their illnesses for an average of 6.1 years (women 5.9, men 6.3 years). Homoeopathic treatment had been applied for an average of 18.6 days (women 18.2, men 18.6 days) prior to emergency admission, and 18 patients had in the past already received homoeopathic treatment of one kind or another.

Table 10.1 Diagnoses established in patients admitted to the ER/ICU of the Medical Department I of the Friedrich-Alexander University Erlangen-Nuremberg April 1995 to March 1996

Indications	*n*		*Receiving homoeopathic treatment*	*n%*
Cardiovascular	1532	44.5%	27	42.9%
Gastrointestinal	817	23.7%	7	11.1%
Pulmonary	534	15.5%	8	12.6%
Neurological	82	2.4%	2	3.2%
Endocrinological metabolic	107	3.1%	1	1.5%
Anaphylaxis	25	0.7%	0	
Sepsis	11	0.3%	0	
Intoxications	95	2.7%	1	1.5%
Electrical accidents	8	0.2%	0	
Transfusion incidents	3	0.08%	0	
Psychosomatic	233	6.7%	17	27%
Total	3447	(100%)	63	(1.87%)

Table 10.2 Indications for homoeopathic treatment in patients with no pathological organic findings at the time of discharge

Diagnosis	*n*
Dyspnoea	4
Anxiety	4
Hyperventilation	7
Affective disorders (multi-chemical syndrome)	3
Supraventricular tachycardia	7
Total	n=25

Table 10.3 Indications for homoeopathic treatment in 63 patients (multiple indications possible)

Indication	*n*	*Indication*	*n*
Glossodynia	5	IBS	4
Asthma	7	Arthrosis	15
Neurodermatitis	3	Chronic fatigue	7
Migraine	12	Infertility	2
Multiple affective disorders	15	Psoriasis	3
Paraesthesia	2	Cystitis	7
Cancer	2	Frequent colds	8
Food allergy	18		

A breakdown of the indications for homoeopathic treatment in the 25 patients is shown in Table 10.3.

Only in nine of the patients was the diagnosis at admission and discharge and the homoeopathic remedy given precisely recorded. Table 10.4 shows the relevant details.

Discussion

We first investigated the question as to whether the presumptive diagnosis on admission established by the care-providing physicians was compatible with the clinical symptoms exhibited by the patient. An analysis of the individual cases showed that at the time of admission, the patients did indeed have appropriate symptoms; thus, patients 1, 3 and 5 actually did suffer from rhythm disorders in the sense of tachycardias or multiple ventricular extrasystoles, and in patients 6 and 7, respiratory distress too was characterized by appropriate subjective symptoms. The subsequent determination of the oxygen content in the blood, however, failed to reveal any partial or global respiratory insufficiency.

It must, however, be noted that the time available to the family doctors, who alone established the diagnosis leading to admission to hospital, was relatively short. The great discrepancy between the diagnosis on admission and diagnosis on discharge may presumably be considered to be the result of wrong diagnoses on the part of the referring physicians.

The question as to whether the establishment of a true diagnosis by the family doctor was at all possible at the time could not be answered. On admission, however, the patients already clearly had dramatic subjective symptoms which, during the stay in hospital, prompted an appropriately careful diagnostic work-up.

A point worth noting is the fact that, in all patients, the diagnosis established was of a psychosomatic nature. The question thus presents itself as to whether patients receiving homoeopathic treatment show a tendency towards mental lability. Such a hypothesis is supported by a number of authors. Thus, in repeated investigations of groups of patients receiving homoeopathic treatment, Furnham and Forey (1994) conclude that these patients significantly suffer more frequently from psychological problems,

Table 10.4 Diagnosis on admission and on discharge; homoeopathic remedies employed in nine patients in an intensive care unit

Patient	*Diagnosis at discharge*	*Diagnosis on admission*	*Indication for homoeopathic therapy*	*Homoeopathic remedy*	*n*	*Gender*	*Age*
1	Psychogenic hyperventilation	Tachycardia Anxiety (state)	Glossodynia	Sulfur X6	1	f	38
2	Autonomic dystonia	Anaphylaxis Agitation	Neurodermatitis	Rhus toxicodendron X200	1	f	41
3	Depression	Supraventricular tachycardia	Arthrosis	Apis X30	1	f	52
4	Depression	Respiratory distress	Migraine	Strontium Carbonicum X100	1	f	39
5	Cardiac neurosis	Cardiac arrhythmias	Food allergy	Nux vomica X100	1	m	47
6	Hyperventilation tetany	Respiratory distress	Rheumatism	Formica X30	1	m	54
7	Hyperventilation tetany	Respiratory distress	Affective disorders	Belladonna X100	1	m	33
8	Anxiety	Myocardial infarction	Psoriasis	Nux vomica X30	1	f	43
9	Neurosis depression	Cerebral haemorrhage	Back pain	Apis X30	1	f	37

and that the locus of control varies. In a study carried out by Hentschel *et al.* (1996), it was shown that these patients have a tendency towards negative affectivity, and require psychotherapeutic treatment significantly more often than the general population.

Another question that needs to be discussed is the extent to which homoeopathic remedies also have toxic effects. In the case of the remedies employed by the patients in the present study, with one exception, the dilutions were above X23.

Assuming that the remedies had been properly prepared, toxicological effects would seem to be excluded. However, such toxicological effects have been reported for Ayurvedic medicine, some constituent(s) of which had contained heavy metals (Keen *et al.*, 1994).

In comparison with the number of patients who had received homoeopathic treatment, which is a relatively small percentage of the overall number of patients (1.9%) studied, the rate of adverse reactions (25 = 39.7%) is relatively high.

Another possible explanation for the symptoms presenting might be nocebo effects. However, reliable relevant data on patients receiving homoeopathic treatment are not available.

Conclusion

In general, undesired clinical events occurring under homoeopathic treatment would appear to be very rare. Nevertheless, these adverse reactions should receive particular attention, and further clinical placebo-controlled studies need to be carried out. Furthermore, adverse reactions following the administration of homoeopathic remedies should be recorded. In the same way as side effects associated with medicaments with confirmed efficacy are recorded (e.g. in Germany by the Federal Institute for Drugs and Medical Products), a clearing centre for adverse reactions associated with homoeopathic remedies should be established in Germany.

References

Aberer, W. and Strohal, R. (1991) Homoeopathic Preparations Severe Adverse Effects, Unproven Benefits. *Dermatologica*, **182** (4), 253.

Benmeir, P., Neumann, A., Weinberg, A., Sucher, E., Welsher, Z., Lusthaus, S., Rotem, M., Ledad, A. and Wechsler, M.R. (1991) Giant Melanoma of Inner Tide: Homoeopathic Life-threatening Negligence. *Ann. Plast. Surg.*, **27** (6), 583–5.

Fischer, P. and Ward, A. (1994) Complementary Medicine in Europe. *British Medical Journal*, **309** (6947), 107–11.

Furnham, A. and Forey, J. (1994) The Attitudes, Behaviours and Beliefs of Patients of Conventional Versus Complementary (Alternative) Medicine. *British Journal of Clinical Psychology*, **50** (3), 458–17.

Hentschel, C., Kohnen, R., Hauser, G., Lindner, M., Hahn, E.G. and Ernst, E. (1996) Complementary Medicine Today: Patients' Decision for Physician or Magician? A Comparative Study of Patients Deciding in Favour of Alternative Therapies. *European Journal of Physical Medicine and Rehabilitation*, **6** (5) (in press).

Keen, R.W., Deacon, A.C. *et al.* (1994) Indian Herbal Remedies for Diabetes as a Cause of Lead Poisoning. *Postgracenal Medical Journal*, **70**, 113–14.

Part IV

Experimental Studies

Chapter 11

Hypothesis of modes of action of homoeopathy: theoretical background and the experimental situation

Fritz-Albert Popp

Introduction

Homoeopathy is an interdisciplinary problem, concerning physics, biology and medicine. Physics, in order to understand the possible modes of action of succussions which do not contain even one molecule of the working substance. Biology, for an explanation of the extraordinary biological sensitivity, including a mechanism that works according to Hahnemann's basic simile, and potency rules. And medicine, playing – apart from statistical analysis of the medical efficacy – the main role in revealing placebo effects and similar phenomena of 'mind-body' interactions.

The physical perspective

Common sense is violated if one postulates that a remedy will work even if not one molecule of the efficient substance is dissolved. Common sense holds that the efficacy of a remedy can be based only on a substantial action, i.e. a molecular interaction of the remedy with a receptor of the patient's body. This dogma has been justified by long experience and scientific work in pharmacology and medicine. We shall note, in addition, that some strange effects like hormesis (Stebbing, 1982) or hormoligosis do not change this point of view, because any effect of any solutions disappears completely as soon as the number of dissolved molecules approaches zero.

It is important to know that even homoeopathy does not doubt this dogma. Rather, the decisive point of homoeopathy is the argument that homoeopathic remedies are not solutions but succussions of the efficient substance (or imprints instead of mixtures in the case of 'globuli').

Now, in the picture that most people have of homoeopathy this argument does not change the situation at all. Again common sense cannot maintain that there is a significant difference between a solution and a succussion. However, this belief is not completely correct. In order to show this, one could, for instance, discuss the obvious case that rather significant differences in the biological effects of cold and hot water arise, although there is certainly no difference in the molecular contents. The decisive difference between cold and hot water is the different distribution of the energy over the molecules (which makes the temperature difference). Let us look in a little more detail into possible differences between solutions and succussions, since this may be a key to understanding homoeopathy. What happens with a fluid if it is succussed? At first, mechanical energy has to be brought up in order to shake up the fluid. For 1g of fluid and 1cm distance of succussions, one needs at least the energy of 9.81erg, corresponding to about 6×10^{12}eV (which is, by the way, 14 orders of magnitude higher than the mean thermal energy kT). Although only a very small amount of this energy really gets stored in the fluid, i.e. by excitation of translational, vibrational, rotational, and electronic states, this extraordinary excitation of excited states usually falls back into the ordinary occupation of the excited states according to the well-known Boltzmann distribution of thermal equilibrium, where with increasing energy E the probability of occupying the states decreases according to $\exp(-E/kT)$. The time between non-thermal excitation of the energy levels and the relaxation into thermal equilibrium is estimated to be about a few nanoseconds, which means that it cannot play any practical role. However, there are conditions which have to be considered a little more carefully in order to get a realistic picture of the complete situation. Needless to say, in addition to the molecular energy levels, some collective states of the fluid are excited. One of the most interesting candidates is, for instance, soliton excitation (Davydov, 1994), which represent 'coherent states' (in the classical picture coherent states are analogues to phase-locked undamped oscillations) with a lot of remarkable properties:

1. There is no doubt today that solitons are excited in water, since solitons have actually been discovered in fluids (water).
2. Solitons manifest non-linear excitation with self-stabilizing properties.
3. Solitons do not interact with thermal phonons, a fact which increases their lifetime considerably.
4. As coherent states, solitons do not decay exponentially, but according to a 1/t law, where t is the time after excitation (Popp and Li, 1993).

Davydov, who investigated solitons very carefully, postulated that solitons are responsible for 'high-temperature-superconductivity' as well as for the well-known extraordinary sensitivity of biological systems (Davydov, 1994). Although these claims are not yet based on solid experimental work, they challenge the opinion that succussions and imprints are completely identical to solutions and mixtures, respectively. Rather, it is very likely that systematic excitations of coherent states by mechanical one-directional shaking prepares some fluids in such a way that a sufficiently long 'memory time' can be obtained provided of course that small enough amplitudes of the coherent oscillations are in effect. Take, for instance, the following realistic example.

The biological system will be about 10^9 times more sensitive than a usual technical detector system working under thermal equilibrium conditions, and the coherent states which are excited in the fluid shall have a 'physical' lifetime t* of 1s which means that their amplitude is damped in such a way that after one second it always drops down to about half of its initial value. Then time t+, within which a biological system can react to the coherent states (which amplitudes after excitation drop down not exponentially but according to a 1/t law), in the fluid is 10^9 times longer than the decay time t* of these collective excitations.

Consequently, the biological system would respond to the original excitation of the fluid even for one hundred years! (corresponding to t+ of about 10^9s) after succusion, in the case that a technical instrument registers a decay time t* of 1s. This realistic example tells us that in spite of the fact that we may register completely uninteresting physical lifetimes of excited states in the order of seconds (within 1s one has no chance to use this memory for practical purposes), biological systems may become aware of them over years, simply in view of their considerably higher sensitivity.

We come to an important conclusion: One cannot exclude the possibility that succussions of fluids are different from solutions in excited coherent states to which a biological system can respond, i.e. in view of:

1 the rather high stability of the coherent state, and
2 the high sensitivity of the biological system compared to technical detector systems.

A serious hypothesis can be distinguished from an unserious one by the fact that it has predictive power which can be examined by critical experiments (these may be also 'thought' experiments). If the physical model described here is correct, one can measure the memory time of water by means of measuring the decay time of excited collective states in water after succussion. There should be a decisive difference in the decay time, registered by physical instruments and the time within which bioindicators can respond to excitation. The prolongation of the decay time (describing the memory effect of water after succussion) could be measured best by non-equilibrium detector systems of high signal/noise ratio and by biological sensors in experiments with high enough statistical reliability.

If it is true that coherent states of long enough lifetime are excited by succussions (or imprints), the required substance-specific modulation of the coherent states by the succussion together with the effective substance is very obvious and does not lead to new, principal problems in understanding the (substance-specific) effects of homoeopathic remedies, even if there is not even one molecule of the substance present any more. Its information is then stored in terms of specific modulations of the spatio-temporal pattern of the coherent oscillations of the fluid (or solid) which work as the carrier waves of the substance-specific modulations (Popp, 1978; 1990).

The biological perspective

Hahnemann's rules for the efficacy of homoeopathy can be reduced to two essential principles:

1 the simile principle, and
2 the potency rule.

The first rule states that the patient has to be treated with that substance which induces just the same symptoms that are characteristic for the disease. The second rule claims that the efficacy is better the 'higher' the potency is, which means that the repetition of succussions under permanent dilution of this substance should be as high as possible. There is no limitation by the

Avogadro's number, i.e. even if no molecule of the effective substance is present any more in the succussion, the potency rule is still valid.

What is important from a scientific point of view is the question of whether both rules are mutually independent or whether the second rule is valid if – and only if – the first rule is satisfied. I discuss only the latter case because if both rules are independently valid, I do not see any possibility of explaining homoeopathy on a scientific basis. In case the potency rule is only valid for the right 'simile', Hahnemann's principles remind us of the resonance phenomenon which is well-known in physics. The more the frequencies of two oscillators agree, the lower the amplitudes necessary for long-range transfer of energy. There is no difference for electric oscillations (e.g. resonance circuit) or for mechanical oscillations (e.g. pendula) or acoustical ones (e.g. tuning forks). Take, for instance, the following simple model. The patient represents a black box in which a series of tuning forks with a variety of different frequencies is oscillating, where one of them (representing the cause of the disease) shall perturb the harmony of all the others by an awkward frequency or frequency combination (while 'disregulating' thereby the regulation pattern of the natural intrinsic oscillations). There is only one way to restore harmony: one has to hang a second tuning fork not too far from the black box (or bring it in) thus taking up by the well-known long-range interaction of resonance a considerable part of the energy of the disregulating oscillating tuning fork in the box (see Figure 11.1). The efficacy is higher, (1) the better the frequency (frequencies) of the added tuning fork fits (fit) with the frequency (frequencies) of the perturbating tuning fork in the interior (simile principle), and (2) the lower the oscillation amplitude of the added tuning fork is before taking up energy from the interior resonating tuning fork (potency rule). There is no doubt that this model is fundamental enough to explain the interaction of coherent states as it is completely consistent with the principles of homoeopathy.

Some scientists object that there is no resonance-like interaction known in biology that is illustrative of Hahnemann's rule. This is not true. One could mention here the vaccination or the Arndt-Schultz rule. However, even more convincing is another well-known but unexplained effect in cell biology. This is the so-called photorepair. High doses of UV light damage the DNA of cells to such an extent that even double-strand breaks occur. Nevertheless, after exposure of the damaged cells to just the same UV light, but now in very small doses, the damage is practically completely repaired within a few hours. Needless to say that this effect works just according to Hahnemann's rules. Substantial interactions are not necessary. In addition, this effect is general for all living cells from single cells up to the entire human body. Although the mechanism is far from being understood, there is no question that we have to develop a deeper understanding of biological functions in order to understand the principles. It is not enough to indicate simply 'molecular interactions', such as, for instance, enzymatic activity. What is then, by the way, the 'regulator' of enzymatic activities? It is impossible that 10^5 reactions per cell and per second regulate themselves by molecular forces. There should actually be interactions (like non-thermal photons from excited states, as, for instance, biophotons) which stabilize the whole system, and it is possible that those governing interactions follow principles such as Hahnemann's rules (corresponding to resonance

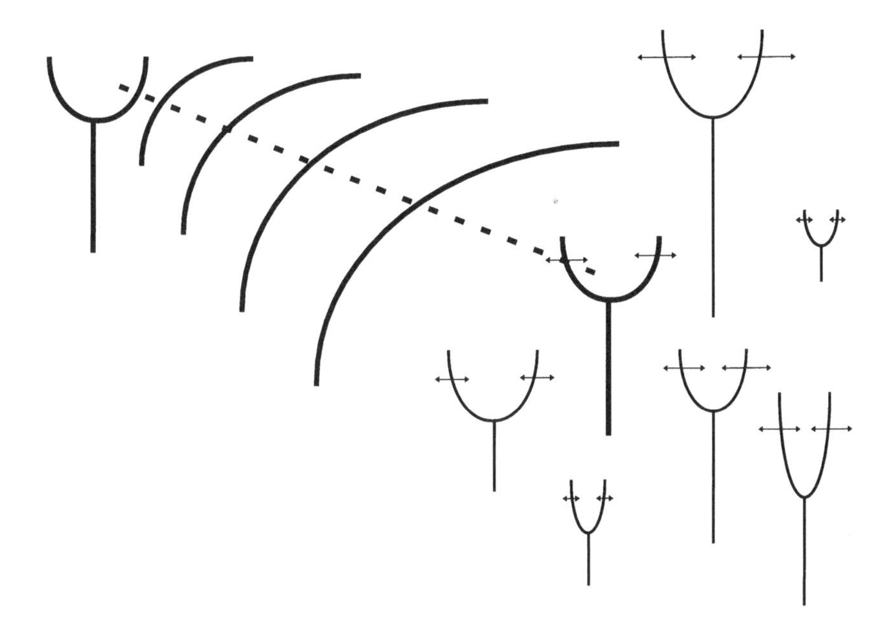

Figure 11.1 The tuning fork model of homoeopathy

phenomena). According to Nicolis and Prigogine, those governing interactions far away from thermal equilibrium could be based only on coherent states (Nicolis and Prigogine, 1977). Our own results on biophoton emission (Popp, Gu and Li, 1994) are in complete agreement with the basic role of coherent states in biological systems, providing thus, in addition, a physical basis of Hahnemann's rules.

This does not mean that there is theoretical or experimental evidence of the efficacy of homoeopathy. However, the consequences of this situation can only be that:

1 Scientists have to confess that there is no serious argument against the principal validity of Hahnemann's rules.
2 Intensive research is necessary to reveal the mechanism of homoeopathy.

I think that the following experimental procedures are most promising: bioindicators should be treated by poisons to such an extent that they develop clear symptoms of poisoning. The same substance (or other substances which induce those symptoms) should be taken for preparing the different succussions of homoeopathy, where all of the possible controls (solvent, succussion of the solvent and the dilution) are always applied in addition to the remedy. It is then only a question of reliable statistics to show experimental evidence of the validity of Hahnemann's rules in biology. I know that it is very difficult to perform those experiments. There are not only scientific reasons which make this kind of research very complicated. However, there is no other way than this, in order to obtain a serious scientific basis for homoeopathy. Fortunately, vastly different fields in modern science are developing in such a way that homoeopathy gets a lot of scientific support by discoveries in other areas, i.e. chaos in biology, new insights into quantum chemistry and solid state physics, but also quantum optics in the non-classical range, where it is well-known nowadays that communication cannot be optimized at the highest, but only at the lowest, number of quanta in a field.

The medical perspective

The question of the efficacy of homoeopathy is one of the most important problems of medicine, because if evidence of homoeopathic efficacy can be shown, modern medicine will certainly change its paradigm, at least it will considerably extend its range. Most mainstream physicians do not reject outright the possibility of homoeopathic efficacy. Their main argument concerns the placebo effect as an explanation of the medical success of homoeopathy.

This argument is serious enough to become the subject of scientific analysis. A placebo effect is the amplification and/or the induction of the patient's healing by his belief in his personal healing. People think that the main reason for this belief is trust in the doctor's help. However, why should trust in the doctor be the only influence to create the placebo effect? Taking account of the fact that this 'belief' is a subjective parameter which cannot be measured, we have to accept that it belongs to a certain state of consciousness displaying a much more general nature, as indicated by, for instance, 'self-confidence' or something similar. We cannot exclude the possibility that this 'belief' or 'self-confidence' can occur as a definite psychological state in children, babies and animals. We have also to accept the possibility that this kind of psychological state is a necessary, even a sufficient condition for any kind of healing or health at all. There is no way to reject all these interconnections between this 'generalized placebo effect' and any kind of interaction between the patient and the treatment.

These necessary considerations – which are to my surprise rarely discussed – lead immediately to a variety of crucial consequences:

1 The placebo hypothesis of homoeopathy can never be rejected with certainty.
2 Even if somebody claimed that allopathic medical success is based on placebo effects, this proposition could not be rejected either.
3 As long as the 'mechanism' of the placebo effect remains unknown, the dismissal of homoeopathy by use of this term discredits the claim, since it shows clearly that it is not a scientific statement.
4 The user of such an argument has to take the responsibility for making homoeopathy unsuccessful by his interference – but only if he were right!

Table 11.1 Belief systems about the basis of homoeopathy

	Physical basis	*Biological basis*	*Medical basis*
Classical medicine	No	No	No
Modern version of classical medicine	No	No	Placebo effects
Biochemistry	No	No	?
Homoeopathy	?	?	Real effect, no placebo effect
Biophysics	No	No	?
Some physicists	Memory effects	Response to 'information' in remedy	?
Observations	Solitons, representatives of coherent states	Resonance-like effects (photorepair)	Interactions of psychological states and health states
Possible scientific point of view	Substance-specific modulated coherent states	Resonance interaction of coherent states	Generalized placebo thesis, based on coherent states

5 The user of such an argument demonstrates his openness for effects which are:

- based only on experience,
- based only on completely 'non-substantial' interactions.

It is difficult to understand why this person would not then believe in homoeopathy.

6 And just the opposite, if somebody requires a substantial interaction for 'real' healing, one would expect that he be open to the possibility that a generalized placebo effect (this means a possibly necessary or even sufficient condition of healing at all!) can be induced also substantially, i.e. by the application of suitable allopathic remedies and, of course, also by homoeopathy according to Hahnemann's rules.

This situation invites us to suggest the following working hypotheses:

a The formation and stabilization of coherent states in the patient's body induce some kind of 'self-confidence', which is a necessary and sufficient condition for any kind of healing.

b Homoeopathic remedies contain coherent states of the carrier media (water-alcohol or sugar) which are modulated substance-specifically by succussion (imprints) with the toxic substance. According to the resonance mechanism of the tuning forks (generally of coherent states) the remedies take up the energy of disregulating coherent states in the patient's body, which are modulated by the corresponding toxic substances. It is evident that this mechanism works just according to Hahnemann's rules.

c The outflow of disregulating energy stabilizes and harmonizes the fundament of the natural body-own coherent states and, as a consequence, induces the necessary and sufficient psychological state of belief in the healing. Whether the patient or/and his observer become aware of this belief is not a decisive factor.

Table 11.1 displays all the arguments again in some kind of brief review.

References

Davydov, A.S. (1994) Energy and Electron Transport in Biological Systems. In *Bioelectrodynamics and Biocommunication* (M.W. Ho, F.A. Popp and U. Warnke, eds) pp. 411–30, World Scientific, London.

Nicolis, G. and Prigogine, I. (1977) *Self-Organization in Non-equilibrium Systems*. A Wiley Interscience Publication, John Wiley & Sons, London.

Popp, F.A. (1978) Deutungsversuche homopathischer Effekte aus moderner physikalischer Sicht. *Allg. Hom. Ztg.*, **223**(46), 93.

Popp, F.A. (1990) Some elements of homeopathy. *British Homoeopathic Journal*, **9**, 161–6.

Popp, F.A. and Li, K.H. (1993) Hyperbolic Relaxation as a Sufficient Condition of a Fully Coherent Ergodic Field. *International Journal of Theoretical Physics,* **32**, 1573–83.

Popp, F.A., Gu, Q. and Li, K.H. (1994) Biophoton Emission: Experimental Background and Theoretical Approaches. *Modern Physics Letters B*, **8**, 1269–96.

Stebbing, A. (1982) Hormesis – The Stimulation of Growth by Low Levels of Inhibitors. *Total Environ.*, **22**, 213–25.

Chapter 12

Theory and experiments on high dilutions

Gerassimos S. Anagnostatos, Polykarpos Pissis, Kyriakos Viras and Maria Soutzidou

Introduction

Homoeopathy claims that a solution of a certain substance even extremely diluted beyond Avogadro's number is effective as a remedy. Although the validity of homoeopathy is still questioned by many, there is a scientific duty to contribute to the resolution of this mystery.

It is apparent that homoeopathic research should be divided into three parts. First, one should test if properties related to the initial substance are carried by the solution even in high dilutions. Second, in case of positive result to the previous test, one should further test if such properties carried by the solution are recognized by the organism receiving the solution. Third, in case of positive results to the previous two tests, one should further test if the reaction of the organism to these properties has any positive or negative effect on the level of health of this organism.

It is apparent that the first test requires physico-chemical study, the second test biological study, and the third test medical study. If any link of the chain made of the above three tests breaks, homoeopathy completely fails. Indeed, if no physico-chemical property is detected that differentiates a homoeopathic solution from the pure solvent in which the mother tincture has been diluted for its preparation, then it becomes meaningless to go on with the study of possible biological and medical effects. Also, what is the meaning in searching for a medical effect if no biological effect exists even if the first test has positive results? In other words the third test is meaningful only if both the previous two tests lead to positive results.

Only the existence of a theory can suggest the specific properties that should be detected (at each step of the research) and for what reasons. Since any homoeopathic remedy is prepared by sequential dilutions of the mother tincture and a number of mechanical impulses applied on each dilution, any successful theory should contain these two basic activities as its necessary ingredients. Also, since it is well known that remedies can be effective either in liquid form or in solid form as lactose tablets, the successful theory should be able to explain this fact as well. Furthermore, since it is well known that homoeopathic remedies are sensitive to high temperatures, that many of them use natural substances as their extracts and that there is a large variety of remedies, the successful theory should be able to explain these properties as well.

The theory (Anagnostatos *et al.*, 1991; Anagnostatos, 1990, 1994) of the present work refers strictly to the physico-chemical study of a remedy, but fortunately is supported by biological studies as well (Sukul, 1992).

In Section 2 the clathrate model is presented, while Sections 3 and 4 describe the experimental support. In Section 5 the results are discussed and finally in Section 6 the conclusions are presented.

The clathrate model

In the present brief presentation of the clathrate model, the tetraisoanylammonium fluoride in water (which may not lead to any homoeopathic remedy) is taken as an example, because the stereochemical structure of its molecule and all details (form and size) of its corresponding clathrate are precisely known (Jeffrey and McMullan, 1967).

In Figure 12.1 all three stages in the preparation of a remedy, according to the clathrate model, are demonstrated and are separated from each other by heavy horizontal lines. In stage one the molecule of the tetra-isoanylammonium fluoride is shown in the centre of Figure 12.1a by bold circles, while the water molecules in the corresponding clathrate are depicted by larger open circles (Jeffrey and McMullan, 1967).

It is apparent that the overall form of the clathrate shape resembles that of the molecule of the mother substance. Even more important is the remark that the three volumes comprising the clathrate are pentagonal dodecahedra, of which two have a common face. This remark holds true for any clathrate, i.e., the building block for all cases of clathrates is the pentagonal dodecahedron (Jeffrey and McMullan, 1967) mainly because of its basic property that its face angle between two adjacent edges of a pentagon (108°) very closely approximates the angle between the two hydrogen atoms in a water molecule. This near coincidence of the above two angles substantially contributes to the necessary strength of the structure of the clathrate made up from such dodecahedra (Stanley, Cook and Castleman, 1990; Yang and Castleman, 1989, 1990).

In Figure 12.1b the second stage in the preparation of a remedy, according to the clathrate model, is demonstrated. During this stage the separation of the molecule of the mother substance from its clathrate, when a forceful mechanical impulse is applied to the dilution, takes place (b_2–b_1). This separation is obtained due to the different inertial kinematic behaviour between the (relatively large density) molecule of the substance and that of the (small density because of the much larger size) clathrate. The inertia of the clathrate is additionally increased due to its connections, via hydrogen bonds, with water molecules of the water layers immediately after the clathrate.

The molecule of the substance at its new, relocated position (b_2) interacts with water molecules and immediately forms a new clathrate identical to the initial one (b_2'). At the same time, the left-over empty clathrate (b_1) acquires a more compact structure than before due to the absence of the hydrophobic repulsive forces between substance and water molecules of the clathrate. Simultaneously, the water molecules of the water layer immediately after the clathrate are affected by the symmetry of the shrunken clathrate

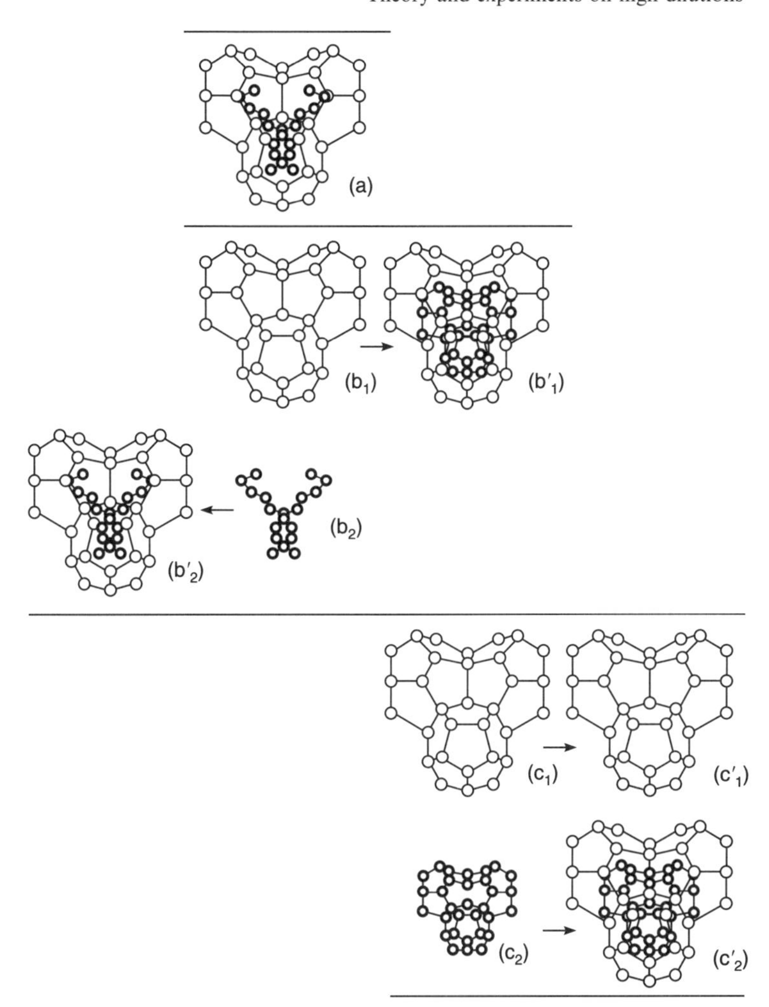

Figure 12.1 Stages in preparing a homoeopathic remedy, where the tetraisoanylammonium fluoride is employed as a hypothetical mother substance for which the molecular stereochemical structure and the corresponding clathrate are precisely known; clathrate (host) formation round the mother substance (guest) after its dilution in water. That is, stereochemical molecular structure of the substance at the centre and clathrate (cage) round it made of water molecules; b_1 and b_2 clathrate and molecule of the substance, respectively, coming from (a) after their separation due to forceful mechanical impulses applied on the solution; b_1' and b_2' evolution of b_1 and b_2 respectively, shortly after the mechanical impulses. Specifically, the mother molecule in b_2 interacts with surrounding water molecules and as a result another clathrate is formed leading to b_2' which is identical to (a). At the same time b_1 shrinks (due to absence of hydrophobic forces with the mother molecule) and interacts with surrounding water molecules and as a result another (mantle) clathrate is formed leading to b_2'. c_1 and c_2 mantle and clathrate, respectively, come from b_1' after their separation due to forceful mechanical impulses applied on the solution. c_1' and c_2' evolution of c_1 and c_2, respectively, shortly after the mechanical impulses. Specifically, the core clathrate in c_2 interacts with surrounding water molecules and as a result another mantle clathrate is formed leading to c_2', which is identical to b_1'. At the same time c_1 shrinks (due to absence of repulsive forces between hydrogen atoms along pairs of parallel edges of the mantle and the core clathrates in b_1') and interacts with surrounding water molecules and as a result another (mantle) clathrate is formed leading to c_1' which is identical to c_2' and b_1'.

(now called core clathrate) and form another clathrate (called mantle clathrate) imitating the shape of the previous clathrate vertex by vertex (b_1'). The mantle clathrate is looser than the core clathrate due to the larger distances between oxygen atoms located at the clathrate corners forming hydrogen bonds along its edges. These distances are further increased due to the repulsive forces between hydrogen atoms of the two clathrates, especially between pairs of hydrogen atoms along pairs of parallel edges of the two clathrates.

In Figure 12.1c the third stage in the preparation of a remedy is presented, where the separation of the core clathrate from its mantle clathrate is obtained, when a forceful mechanical impulse is applied on the dilution (c_2 and c_1). This is possible due to the different inertial kinematic behaviour between the compact core clathrate (behaving like a solid) and the loose mantle clathrate (behaving like a liquid with an increased viscosity), whose inertia is additionally increased due to its connections, via hydrogen bonds, with water molecules of the water layers immediately after the mantle clathrate.

The core clathrate at its new, relocated position (c_2) interacts with water molecule and almost immediately forms a new mantle clathrate identical to the initial mantle clathrate (c_2'). The left-over empty clathrate (c_1) acquires a more compact structure than before, because, due to the absence of the core clathrate, shorter distances between oxygen atoms at the vertices of the clathrate are permitted. Simultaneously the water molecules of the water layer immediately after the clathrate are affected by the symmetry of the shrunken clathrate (now becoming core clathrate) and form another (mantle) clathrate imitating the shape of the previous clathrate vertex by vertex (c_1'). This new mantle clathrate is identical to the mantle clathrates of $b_1' - c_2'$.

An essential feature of the model is the assumed stability of clathrates (filled or empty). Theoretical and experimental studies (Stanley, Cook and Castleman, 1990; Yang and Castleman, 1989, 1990) however, lend support to this assumption. It is finally going to be tested simultaneously with the experimental efforts to detect possible physico-chemical properties of homoeopathic preparations.

According to the clathrate model, the final outcome of the sequential dilutions and mechanical impulses applied during the preparation of a homoeopathic remedy is a coexistence of molecules of the mother substance surrounded by their clathrates and of empty core clathrates surrounded by their mantle clathrates.

As the number of sequential dilutions increases, the molecules of the mother substance become more and more rare. Practically speaking, after the dilutions overpass Avogadro's number, these molecules have an almost zero probability of appearance. Thus, effectively for high dilutions only core clathrates with their mantle clathrates and, of course, unaffected (free, bulk) water molecules exist.

In other words, in high dilutions there are two water phases, the one made of free water molecules and the other of water molecules bound in structures of clathrates. Thus, experimental techniques distinguishing free from bound water molecules (e.g. dielectric measurements) or techniques detecting change of phase occurring, for example, during heating of the remedy (e.g. differential scanning calorimetric measurements) are appropriate for testing the clathrate model.

Dielectric measurements

Dielectric methods are very powerful in hydration studies. They make use of the different dielectric relaxation time τ of hydration water molecules compared to that of free water molecules due to disturbance of their microdynamics by the solute molecules.

It has been pointed out previously (Pissis, Diamanti and Boudouris, 1983) that one may avoid problems in the analysis of the measurements by using the depolarization thermocurrent (DTC) method. In the DTC method the measurements have to be carried out in frozen solutions at subzero temperatures. For interpretation, the results of these measurements have to be compared with those of DTC measurements in pure ice.

The DTC method is as follows (Bucci, Fieschi and Guidi, 1966; Vanderschueren and Gasiot, 1979). The sample is polarized by an applied electric field E_p at a temperature T_p. This polarization is subsequently frozen in by cooling the sample to a temperature T_o sufficiently low to prevent depolarization by thermal energy. The field is then switched off and the sample is warmed at a constant rate b, while the depolarization current is detected by an electrometer. In the case of a single relaxation process obeying the Arrhenius equation $\tau(T) = \tau_o \times \exp(W/K_B T)$, the depolarization current density J(T) is given by Equation 1.

$$J(T) = (P_o/\tau_o)\exp(-W/k_B T) \times \exp\left(-\frac{1}{b\tau_o}\int_{T_o}^{T} \exp(-W/k_B T')dT'\right), \qquad (1)$$

where τ is the relaxation time, W the activation energy of the relaxation, τ_o the pre-exponential factor, T the absolute temperature, k_B Boltzmann's constant, and P_o the initial polarization. The analysis of the shape of this curve makes it possible to obtain the activation energy W, the pre-exponential factor τ_o, and the contribution $\Delta\varepsilon$ of the peak to the static permittivity (Bucci, Fieschi and Guidi, 1966; Vanderschueren and Gasiot, 1979).

The DTC apparatus (of the National Technical University of Athens) used in the present study consisted of a cryostat, in which the sample temperature could be varied from 77 to 400K, at heating rates between 0.8 and 15Kmin^{-1}. The measuring capacitor was made of brass. The sample temperature was measured by a copper-constantan thermocouple attached to the upper (grounded) electrode. The current was measured with a Keithley 610C electrometer and recorded, simultaneously with the temperature of the sample, with a YEW 3083 XY recorder. The temperature was controlled by a Barber-Colman 520 controller.

We repeatedly performed dielectric measurements on several samples rather shortly after their preparation. The samples were chamomile extract

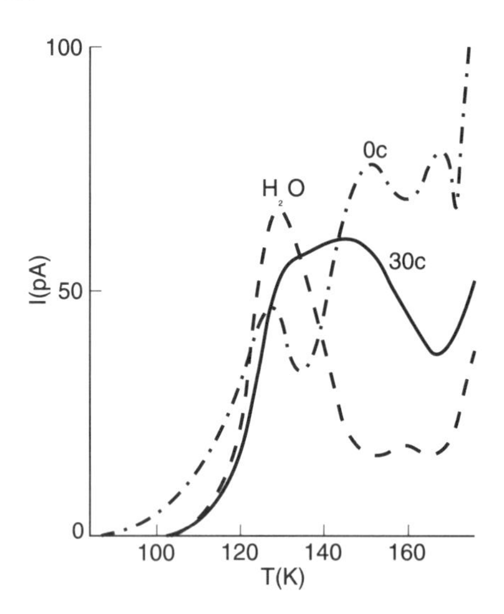

Figure 12.2 Dielectric measurements plots for chamomile-extract water solutions of 0c and 30c dilutions together with the reference plot for water.

prepared by exclusive use of de-ionized, double distilled water at room temperature (i.e. no alcohol was used at any stage of their preparation).The dilutions employed were 0c, 1c, 6c, 12c and 30c, where c denotes that centesimal dilutions were used (i.e. each new dilution was obtained by adding one drop of the previous dilution into 99 drops of doubly distilled, de-ionized water and then applying a number of forceful mechanical impulses) and 0, 1, 6, 12 and 30 stand for an identification of the mother tincture (here chamomile extract) and the first, sixth, twelfth and thirtieth dilution.

The results of dielectric measurements were positive for all samples in the sense that a substantial percentage of bound water molecules was detected in all cases as shown in Figures 12.2 and 12.3, and discussed below.

Figure 12.2 presents three curves labelled H_2O, 0c and 30c. The H_2O curve stands for DTC measurements of pure water and its characteristic peak at about 130K is used as a reference for the other two curves and, in general, for any other curve derived from such measurements as, for example, those shown in Figure 12.3.

The 0c curve in Figure 12. 2 stands for DTC measurements of the mother tincture (here chamomile extract). It is noticeable that its peak at about 130°K presenting unbound water (since its temperature roughly coincides with that of the reference peak for unbound, pure water in the H_2O curve) is shorter (it corresponds to less pA) than the second peak (at about 150°K presenting bound water (since it does not appear at all in the reference curve H_2O for unbound water). This difference in the height of the two peaks means that a greater percentage of water molecules are bound than unbound in the extract of the mother tincture. This, of course, is not surprising since in our dense chamomile extract many water molecules, for instance in the form of clathrate hydrates, are bound (i.e. they have restricted motion

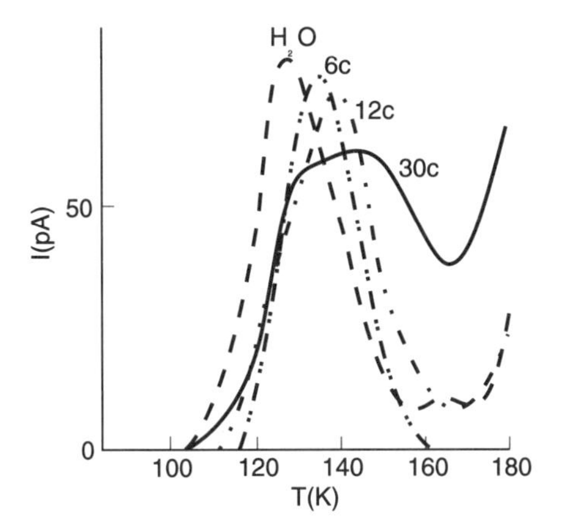

Figure 12.3 Dielectric measurements plots for chamomile-extract water solutions of 6c, 12c and 30c dilutions. Going from lower to higher dilutions, a shift of the plot to higher temperature is noticeable.

with respect to molecules far apart from 'impurity' – chamomile origin – molecules).

The 30c curve stands for similar measurements of the homonymous dilution. Again, like the 0c curve, two peaks appear at about 130K and 150K. The first stands for unbound water and the second for bound water in slightly higher percentage. Additional peaks at different temperatures in all three parts of Figure 12.2 are not meaningful in the present discussion. The basic meaning of Figure 12.2 is that a large percentage of bound to free water molecules exist in the dense 0c solution, where there are many 'impurity' molecules coming from chamomile, but also in the 30c solution where effectively there is not even one 'impurity' molecule. This important conclusion is consistent with the predictions of the clathrate model (Anagnostatos *et al.*, 1991; Anagnostatos, 1990, 1994), where the 'impurity' molecule and the core clathrate can form new clathrates during the application of mechanical impulses on the solution.

Figure 12.3 also presents three curves labelled 6c, 12c and 30c whose notations have already been explained. Two main conclusions could be drawn from this figure. One is that the peak of bound water, relative to the peak of free (unbound) water, is more pronounced for the lower dilutions in such a way that the free water peak can hardly be seen in the curve 6c. This could be thought of as related to the presence of molecules coming from chamomile which increase as we go to lower and lower dilutions. The presence of such molecules in lower dilutions makes the creation of new water formation, during the application of forceful mechanical impulses, on each solution more and more efficient. Of course, more and more water formations (e.g. in the form of clathrates) means more and more bound water molecules. The reason for observing bound water molecules in the dilutions 12c and 30c apparently has no relationship to molecules coming from the chamomile extract which, for these dilutions, are practically zero. The appearance of bound water in these dilutions, however, is explained by the clathrate model (Anagnostatos *et al.*, 1991; Anagnostatos, 1990, 1994).

The second remark is that the peak of bound water shifts more to the right (i.e. to higher temperatures) as we go to higher dilutions. This could be attributed to the creation of stronger water formations, made of bound water molecules, for example in the form of clathrates, as we go to higher and higher dilutions. Such a possibility is permissible in the framework of the clathrate model as has been discussed (Anagnostatos *et al.*, 1991; Anagnostatos, 1990, 1994).

By assuming hydrophobic forces between water and molecules coming from chamomile, water molecules are bound among themselves via hydrogen bonds and form a filled clathrate around each chamomile molecule (like that presented by Figure 12.1a–b'_2), which is energetically weaker than an empty clathrate formed by water molecules alone (like that presented by Figure 12.1c_2). This is reasonable, since the absence of hydrophobic forces in the case of an empty clathrate makes the corresponding structure stronger.

However, another possible reason for an increased stability of water formations in high dilutions is the presence of a huge number of clathrates in these solutions. Indeed, when the number of clathrates is substantial with respect to the number of free water molecules, extra hydrogen bonds may occur among the clathrates themselves. Such extra bonds increase the percentage of bound to free water molecules and also the average stability of water formations. Thus, a solution resulting from a certain large number of sequential dilutions (which has a huge number of empty clathrates) may exhibit an increased average stability of water formations. Indeed, such a prediction, according to the clathrate model, is consistent with the results of our dielectric measurements on high dilutions of chamomile extract.

Hence, all experimental findings coming from our dielectric measurements are consistent with the predictions of the clathrate model.

Differential scanning calorimetric measurements

The differential scanning calorimetry (DSC) measures the amount of energy which is absorbed or released from a sample during its heating or cooling, or when the sample is maintained at a constant temperature (Atwood, Davies and MacNicol, 1991). Thus, any change of phase of a material can be studied in the temperature range from 77 to 900K. In the case of solutions, the heat of each dilution ΔH, its dependence from the temperature, the thermal capacity of solutions and their mixing entropy can be calculated. The apparatus (of the Kapodistrian University of Athens) used in our experiments was a Perkin Elmer DSC-4 model.

We have repeatedly performed differential scanning calorimetric measurements on the same samples with those used in dielectric measurements. That is, we used again chamomile extract of 0c, 1c, 6c, 12c and 30c dilutions. The results of our DSC measurements were positive for all samples in the sense that a change of phase was observed in all cases (Figure 12.4). This change of phase, according to the clathrate model, implies the destruction of the clathrate structures around a certain temperature. It

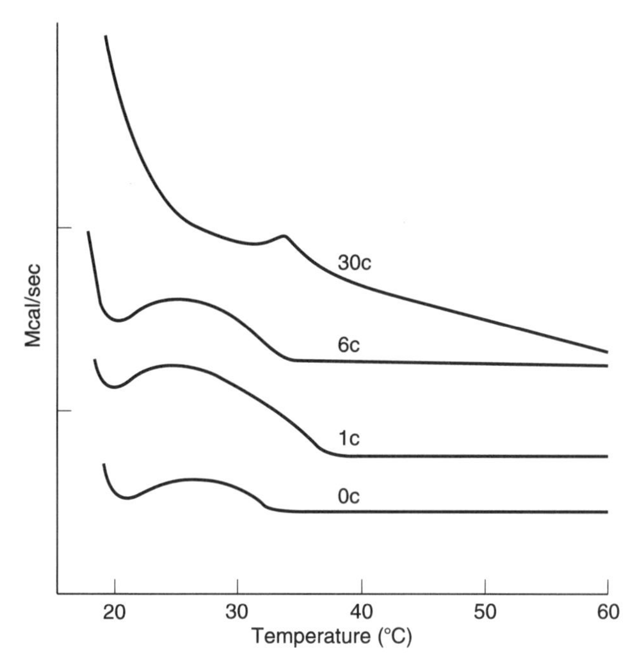

Figure 12.4 Differential scanning calorimetric plots for chamomile-extract water solutions of 0c, 1c, 6c and 30c dilutions.

is noticeable that this temperature shows a small shift to higher values as we proceed from low to high dilutions. This shift reminds one of the similar shift observed in the dielectric measurements discussed above and, according to the clathrate model, has the same explanation.

By using the DSC technique the following two additional series of experiments were performed. The first was a repetition of the previous experiments on the same sequential dilutions of chamomile extract but without applying any mechanical impulse on any dilution. For all dilutions no detectable effect was observed. Thus, mechanical impulses are absolutely necessary for the appearance of a measurable physico-chemical effect. Of course, in up to 12c dilutions some molecules (and their clathrates) coming from the chamomile extract are present, but there are not enough of them for a sizeable (detectable) effect when using the DSC technique. The mechanical impulses, according to the clathrate model, multiply the number of clathrates and make their effect detectable.

The other additional series was a repetition of the same experiments but using de-ionized, double distilled water as mother substance in the place of chamomile extract and applying again a number of mechanical impulses on each dilution. That is, the 1c dilution is obtained by adding one drop of de-ionized, double distilled water into 99 drops of the same water and then applying a number of mechanical impulses (the same as previously) on this dilution. The higher dilutions are also obtained by following the standard approach, that is each dilution is obtained by taking one drop of the previous dilution and adding this drop into 99 drops of double distilled water and

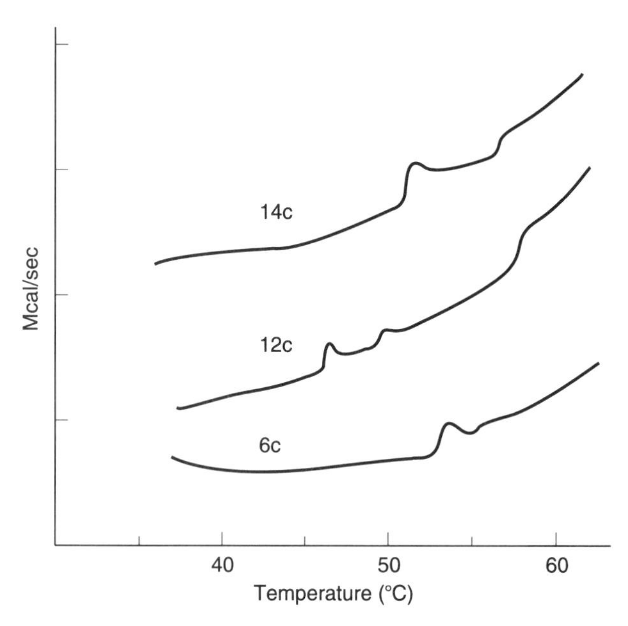

Figure 12.5 Differential scanning calorimetric plots for methanol (CH_3-OH) water solutions of 6c, 12c and 14c dilutions.

then applying the same number of mechanical impulses as before. For all dilutions (i.e. 0c, 1c, 6c, 12c and 30c) again no effect was observed. Thus, the presence of a mother substance for the preparation of a high dilution is essential, a fact which is also consistent with the predictions of the clathrate model, according to which the initial (full) clathrates are formed round the molecules of the mother substance (see Figure 12.1a–b$'_2$), which specifies the kind of clathrates formed. Without these initial clathrates no further clathrates can be formed.

Another series of DSC experiments was performed by employing methanol (CH_3–OH) as mother substance in the place of chamomile extract. All other parameters were kept the same as for the experiments described above. Again the results were positive with respect to the predictions of the clathrate model. That is, again a change of phase is observed at a certain temperature, where according to the model a destruction of the clathrate structures occurs (Figure 12.5). However, it is not clear here if an upward shift of this characteristic temperature occurs by going from lower to higher dilutions, as it has clearly been noticed in the chamomile DSC experiments.

What is important in this series of experiments is the difference, with respect to the chamomile experiments, in the characteristic temperature where we observe the change of phase. That is, while this temperature is about 24°C for the chamomile extract, it is about 52°C for the methanol. This difference in temperature constitutes a further justification of the clathrate model. Indeed, for a different mother substance, a different clathrate is expected which, in general, requires a different amount of heat in order to be destroyed. Since all masses involved in the experiment are kept constant (i.e. the same masses for the chamomile extract and for the methanol experiments), the different amount of heat necessary for the destruction of the different clathrates involved corresponds to different temperature.

In Figure 12.5 we observe two instead of one peak for the 12c dilution. While many other explanations could exist, the following is a plausible one. That is, the initial water formation (clathrate) is transformed during the procedure of preparation or of heating into two simpler (and thus probably thermally weaker) clathrate structures. Each of these two structures is sensitive at its own temperature.

Finally, a preliminary experiment was done for another 1c dilution by using agaricus muscaricus as mother tincture. Again a change of phase is observed and this time at a temperature which is different to both characteristic temperatures observed above for the previously described chamomile and methanol experiments. Indeed, this characteristic temperature of change of phase constitutes a way to differentiate among high dilutions of different substances.

Hence, all differential scanning calorimetric findings are consistent with the predictions of the clathrate model and also with the previous findings of dielectric measurements.

Compressibility, positron annihilation, dielectric, ultrasonic, nuclear magnetic resonance, refractive index, density, viscosity, neutron scattering and X-ray scattering measurements in several alcohol-water mixtures show that there is a critical alcohol mole fraction for which all water is involved in water clusters around alcohol molecules (Jerie *et al.*,1987; Tabellout *et al.*, 1990; Fioretto *et al.*, 1992; Petrillo, Onori and Facchetti, 1989). For alcohol mole fractions lower than the critical one, the number of water molecules involved in clusters increases with increasing alcohol concentration. The following work is restricted to methanol mole fractions lower than the critical one.

The purpose of this study is twofold. (a) To show that the multiplication of water clusters by increasing the alcohol concentration can be shown in a differential scanning calorimetry (DSC) thermogram. (b) To show that a similiar multiplication can be obtained by applying mechanical impulses on a given concentration of alcohol-water mixture. Apparently, the number of clusters beyond the number of methanol molecules are hole water clusters containing no methanol molecules in their interior.

For the realization of objective (a) mixtures of 0.02 and 0.04 methanol mole fractions were used. For the realization of objective (b) mechanical impulses were applied on a mixture of 0.02 methanol mole fraction.

Thermogram (a) in Figure 12.6 refers to a 0.02 methanol mole fraction. Thermogram (b) refers to a 0.04 methanol mole fraction. By comparing thermograms (a) and (b) it is apparent that the higher concentration exhibits higher peaks, i.e. the number of clusters increases with increasing methanol concentration. This observation is consistent with the interpretation given concerning the nature of the DSC peak around 52°C, that refers to water clusters around methanol molecules.

Thermogram (c) in Figure 12.6 shows the multiplication of the number of clusters (higher DSC peak) included by applying mechanical impulses on a mixture of 0.02 methanol mole fraction. Mechanical impulses are here obtained by exposing the mixture for 30 seconds to supersonic waves of frequency 20kHz and power 20Watt. Thus, mechanical impulses lead to

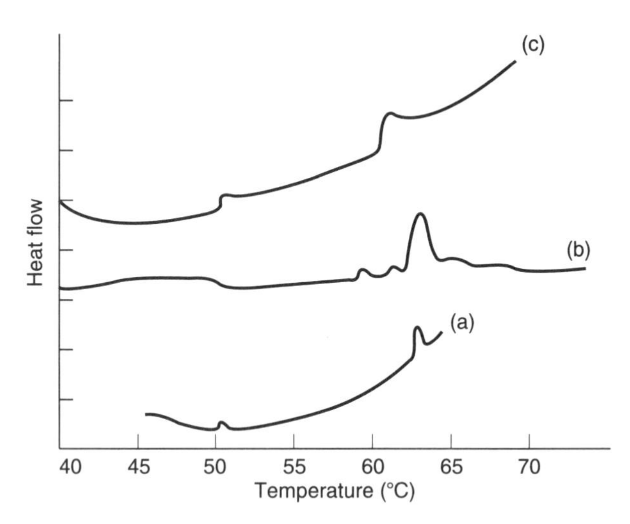

Figure 12.6 DSC thermograms of methanol-water solution for (a) 0.002 mole fraction of methanol (b) 0.004 mole fraction of methanol (c) 0.002 mole fraction of methanol exposed to supersonic waves.

the formation of additional water clusters, which are also stable in thermodynamic equilibrium in the water environment and are destroyed at about the same temperature with the initial clusters.

As known each cluster of water molecules in the methanol-water mixture is formed around the CH_3^- group which constitutes the hydrophobic part of the methanol molecule CH_3OH, while the OH^- group, which constitutes the hydrophilic part of this molecule, participates in the cluster contributing to its stability (Bulone *et al.*, 1989).

Through the mechanical impulses induced multiplication of water clusters, we arrived at water clusters containing no methanol molecule, which are also stable without the absence of the OH^- group to be critical for their stability.

Discussion of the results

The experimental findings of the present study have been presented on pp. 157–64. It has been shown that there is experimental support for the proposed clathrate model that homoeopathic remedies exhibit a structure, which differentiates them from the properties of their solvent. This support comes from two independent experimental techniques and by using two different mother tinctures. Indeed, both of these techniques and both of the mother tinctures employed support the existence of clathrates in remedies made of water molecules interacting via hydrogen bonding. These clathrates constitute a different phase of water than the bulk water. A change of phase from clathrate water to bulk water occurs at specific temperature which is characteristic of the specific clathrates formed and thus of the specific mother tincture used as solute.

Furthermore, necessary conditions for the creation of clathrates, and thus for the preparation of a remedy, are the existence of a mother tincture and the application of mechanical impulses on each dilution. The use of sequential dilutions is a necessity for obtaining dilutions beyond Avogadro's number and for obtaining more stable clathrate structures by increasing the density of clathrates and their interaction which leads to clusters of clathrates.

Extracts from natural sources usually have hydrophobic parts in their molecular structure which are necessary for creation of clathrates. Different natural sources (their extracts) apparently lead to different (in form and size) clathrates with different dielectric and thermal behaviour able to differentiate among the different remedies produced by their extracts.

Finally, we could remark that the structure and stability of clathrates permit the existence (up to a certain temperature) of clathrates on the surface (exterior and interior) of lactose when the remedy is supplied in a solid form. Specifically, when the liquid remedy is poured on the lactose, the molecules of the free (bulk) water eventually evaporate at any temperature, while the bound water molecules in the form of clathrates remain on the lactose as long as the temperature is below a certain value characteristic of relevant clathrate. Later on, when the lactose enters into the organism, the clathrates eventually are mixed with the surrounded liquids of the organism.

Conclusions

In the present study a theory and its experimental (Anagnostatos, Pissis and Viras, 1993) support was presented that the physico-chemical properties of a homoeopathic remedy are different from those of the relevant solvent. These findings give substance to the homoeopathic remedy even at dilutions beyond Avogadro's number.

In general, properties of homoeopathic preparations found in the experiments here employed are consistent with all basic empirically known properties of homoeopathic remedies.

Finally, we can say that new experiments by using the same and additional techniques and a variety of mother tinctures are urgently needed before a definite conclusion is drawn concerning the nature of homoeopathic remedies.

References

Anagnostatos, G.S. (1990) Water small clusters (clathrates) in homoeopathy. Proceeding of the 8th International Conference on the Physics of Thin Films, Kiev, USSR, May.

Anagnostatos, G.S. (1994) Small water clusters (clathrates) in the preparation process of homoeopathy. In: P.C. Endler and J. Schulte, eds. *Ultra high dilution*. Dordrecht: Kluwer Academic Publishers, 121–8.

Anagnostatos, G.S., Pissis, P. and Viras, K. (1993) Proceedings of the 2nd International Conference on Atomic and Nuclear Clusters '93, p. 215, Santorini, Greece, 28 June.

Anagnostatos, G.S., Vithoulkas, G., Garzonis, P. and Tavouxoglou, C. (1991) A working hypothesis for homoeopathetic microdiluded remedies. *The Berlin Journal on Research in Homoeopathy*, **1**, 141–7.

Atwood, J.L., Davies, J.E.D. and MacNicol (1991) *Inclusion Compounds.* Oxford University Press, Oxford.

Bucci, C., Fieschi, R. and Guidi, G. (1966) Ionic thermocurrents in dielectrics. *Physical Review,* **148**, 816–23.

Bulone, D., Spinnato, C., Madonia, F. and Palma, M.U. (1989) *J. Chem. Phys.,* **91**, 408.

Fioretto, D., Marini, A., Onori, G., Palmieri, L., Santucci, A., Socino, G. and Verdini, L. (1992) *Chem. Phys. Lett.* **196**, 583.

Jeffrey, G.A. and McMullan, R.K. (1967) The clathrate hydrates and references therein. *Progress in Inorganic Chemistry,* **8**, 43–107.

Jerie, K., Baranowski, A., Rozenfeld, B., Glinski, J. and Ernst, S. (1987) *Physica Scripta,* **35**, 729.

Petrillo, C., Onori, G. and Facchetti, S. (1989) *Mol. Phys.*, **67**, 697.

Pissis, P., Diamanti, D. and Boudouris, G. (1983) Depolarisation thermocurrents in frozen aqueous solutions of glucose. *Journal of Physics,* **D16**, 1311–22.

Sopev, A.K. and Finney, J.L. (1993) *Phys. Rev. Lett.*, **71**, 4346.

Stanley, R.J., Cook, M. and Castleman, A.W. Jr. (1990) Unimolecular dissociation rate constants: chlorobenzene cations revisited by using a new method. *Journal of Physics Chemistry,* **94**, 3668–74.

Sukul, N.C. (1992) Mechanical Agitation, the Main Factor in Increasing the Efficacy of Agaricus muscarius. A Homoeopathic Drug. *Enviroment and Ecology,* **10**, 7–10.

Tabellout, M., Lanceleur, P., Emery, J.R., Hayaward, D. and Rethrick, R.A. (1990) *J. Chem. Soc. Faraday Trans.*, **86**, 1493.

Vanderschueren, J. and Gasiot, J. (1979) Field-induced thermally stimulated currents. In: *Topics in Applied Physics, 37: Thermally stimulated relaxation in solids*, P. Braunlich, ed. Springer, Berlin, 135–223.

Yang, X. and Castleman, A.W. Jr. (1989) Large protonated water clusters $H^+(H_2O)_n$ ($1 \leq n > 60$): the production and reactivity of clathrate-like structures under thermal conditions. *Journal of the American Chemical Society,* **111,** 6845–6.

Yang, X. and Castleman, A.W. Jr. (1990) Production and magic numbers of large hydrated anion clusters $X^-(H_2O)_{n=0-59}$($X = OH, O, O_2$, and O_3) under thermal conditions. *Journal of Physical Chemistry,* **94**, 8500–502.

Chapter 13

Biochemical studies of the development of the effect of selected homoeopathic agents – in vivo and in vitro models

Günther Harisch and Joachim Dittmann

Introduction

The scientific value or lack of value of homoeopathy can only be assessed on the basis of existing data obtained with the spectrum of methods used in the natural sciences. Without establishing or being able to establish a connection with such data, views on this matter are without reliable value.

The acquisition of this data must be carried out in a speciality-related way. This practice which is useful and therefore customary in other scientific fields should be followed in homoeopathy research as well. In this way, a division of the necessary research into the following two types naturally results:

- Research on the medicament which can be carried out within the context of physics or physical and analytical chemistry.
- Research on the development of the effect with regard to biomolecules and biological functions which can be carried out within the context of biochemistry, physiology and pharmacology.

Using clinical-therapeutic studies, it is not possible to carry out causal research in the sense of proving or rejecting the view that homoeopathy is based on the laws of nature. Therefore, clinical studies can only be regarded as an addition to basic research. With this realization, the normal and sensible way of proceeding in traditional medicine is simply being applied to homoeopathy research as well. On the basis of these considerations, there can be no 'homoeopathy research', but rather a homoeopathic area of scientific research.

Development of the effects of selected homoeopathic agents with regard to biomolecules and biologically relevant functions

In this chapter, only those experiments can be considered which can be profitably carried out using the methods of biochemistry. Research on medicaments cannot be carried out with biochemical methods.

Suitable in vivo (Dittmann and Harisch, 1993; Groß, 1994; Harisch and Kretschmer, 1990; Harisch, Kretschmer and Riemann-Gürlich, 1992a,b; Hentges, 1994; Kretschmer and Harisch, 1992; Theenhaus, Dittmann and Harisch, 1993, 1995) and in vitro models (Dittmann and Harisch, 1994, 1995, 1996a,b,c; Dittmann, Hentges and Harisch, 1994; Dittmann, Selbach *et al.*, 1994; Then *et al.*, 1996a,b) are available for these biochemical studies. The results obtained with these two alternatives should be differently evaluated.

Importance of in vivo experiments

As a rule, the test substance is administered orally or parenterally to rats as experimental animals. Its effect usually develops first in the entire organism by way of several different functional systems, then in the organs, organ cells, and finally in the subcellular organelles. A measurement quantity as parameter is arbitrarily chosen from the series of functions involved.

Due to the uninfluenced development of the effect throughout the entire organism, the result obtained is biologically relevant. Superficially, this appears to be an advantage. However, no direct causal connection between the applied substance and the effect can be established because, as a rule, the quantity of the substance administered is not sufficient for this.

Here however it is not only a case of the lack of a clear quantitative relationship between substance and effect, but above all of the indirectness of the relationship. In other words, with in vivo experiments, the lawfulness of the influence exerted by a particular biomolecule cannot be recognized with sufficient precision.

However, knowledge of the lawfulness of this relationship is indispensable for the resolving of all questions involving homoeopathy.

The in vitro experiment remedies and clarifies matters.

Importance of in vitro experiments

This can involve experiments with cell cultures (Then *et al.*, 1996a,b) or studies on cell-free systems (Dittmann and Harisch, 1994, 1995, 1996a,b,c; Dittmann, Hentges and Harisch, 1994; Dittmann, Selbach *et al.*, 1994). Due to fundamental advantages, only cell-free systems should come under consideration.

In this case, a particular isolated biomolecule comes in contact with the test substance under suitable conditions and the two can react with one another (Figure 13.1). Thus, the type of influence exerted on the molecule can be investigated. It can also be a case of no influence being exerted.

With these experiments, a clear causal connection can be made between test substance and biomolecule. However, it cannot be determined whether the interaction would proceed in the same way or some other way under in vivo conditions (see above).

The results obtained with in vitro experiments need not agree with those obtained for the entire organism. This disadvantage is more than

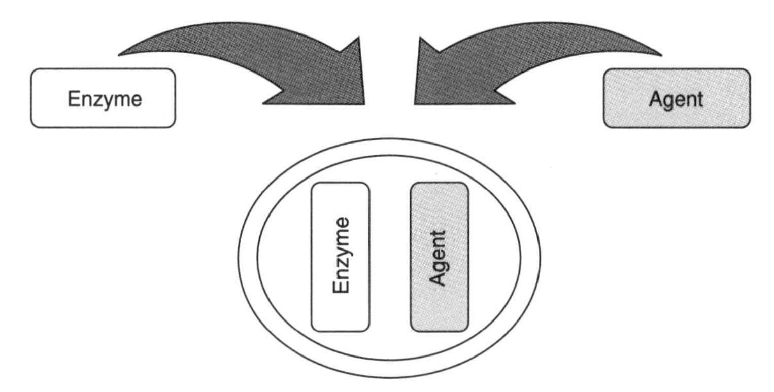

Figure 13.1 Schematic diagram of a cell-free system.

compensated for by the clear advantage of the recognizable causal connection.

Reductionism has a price, but it also offers an opportunity.

Sequence of in vivo and in vitro experiments

Based on the above-mentioned connections, it is reasonable to carry out the in vitro experiment after the in vivo experiment and not vice versa. An overall view depends on the availability of both types of results.

Special features inherent in homoeopathy

Homoeopathy research must take into account the fact that homoeopathic agents are produced by a special procedure referred to as potentization.

Starting with a stock solution, referred to as the mother tincture, consecutive 1:10 or 1:100 steps are employed to produce the desired final attenuation, also referred to as potency. Between the attenuation steps, trituration (milk-sugar preparations) or succussion (ethanol-water preparations) is also stipulated.

Normally, dilutions of a substance are brought to the desired final concentration in one step without having to follow any special procedures – at most, normal laboratory procedures and in this respect not familiar to everyone.

This fact implies that two types of 'attenuations' are required for the investigation of the development of effects of homoeopathic agents:

- The potency produced in accordance with homoeopathic guidelines.
- Conventional dilution of the active substance concerned which must, however, show the same active substance quantity as the potency.

The correspondence between the concentrations can be tested up to the detection limit for the substance involved. Over and above that, testing is

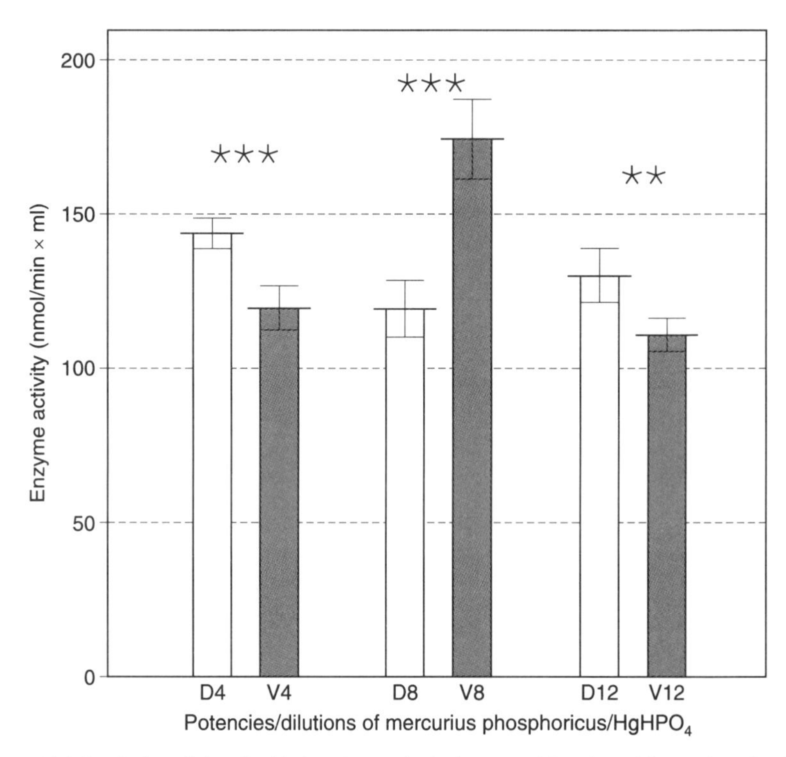

Figure 13.2 Catalytic activity of acid phosphatase in the lysosomal fraction. After oral application of mercurius phosphoricus potencies (D4, D8, D12) or $HgHPO_4$ dilutions (10^{-4} (V4), 10^{-8} (V8), 10^{-12} (V12) over a period of seven days, the rats (male Charles River Wistar rats) were decapitated and their livers removed. Activity of acid phosphatase was determined in the lysosomal fraction obtained by several centrifugation steps of liver homogenate. Significant differences between potency and corresponding dilution are indicated by asterisks (**: $p < 0.01$; ***: $p < 0.001$).

not possible. Testing is also not possible, or at most possible on a selective basis, with botanical homeopathic agents because of the multitude of substances contained in them.

Results from in vivo studies on functional parameters

It could be recognized with this experimental design that the characteristics of the development of the effect are non-linear (Harisch, Kretschmer and Riemann-Gürlich, 1992a,b; Dittmann and Harisch, 1993).

This non-linear dose–effect relationship is expressed in two opposing tendencies. The first possibility exhibits the following characteristics:

- The direct or indirect (see above) influence of the orally administered active substance on a functional parameter (subcellular enzyme) decreases up to a particular potency only to increase again with higher potencies (Figure 13.2) (Harish, Kretschmer and Riemann-Gürlich, 1992b).

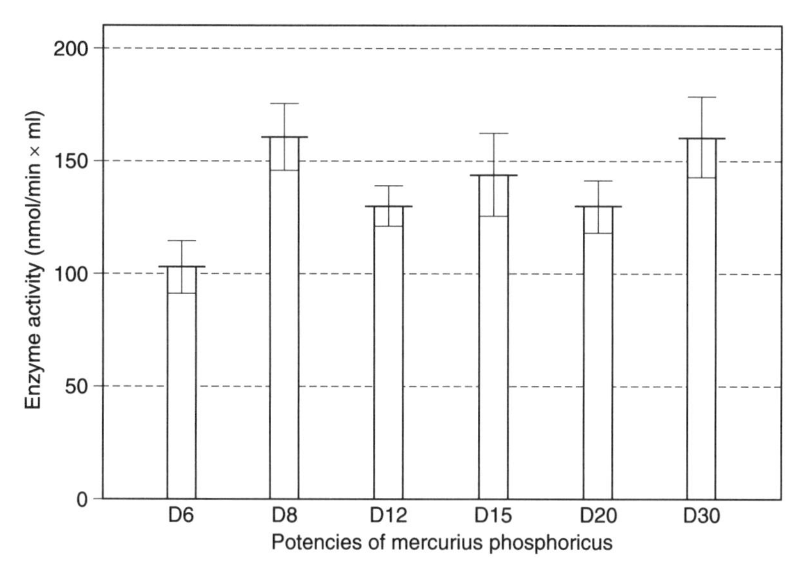

Figure 13.3 Activity of cytochrome c-oxidase. The catalytic activity of this enzyme was determined in the mitochondrial fraction of liver homogenate isolated from male rats which were administered mercurius phosphoricus potencies in dilution steps indicated above over a period of three days.

The second possibility is diametrically opposed to the first:

- The influence of the active substance administered on a parameter increases up to a particular potency only to decrease again with higher potencies (Figure 13.3).

The effect characteristics obtained for conventional dilution are in the same direction but on a lower or higher level. However, they can also be in the opposite direction (Figure 13.4) (Hentges, 1994).

Results from in vivo studies on structural parameters

The influence on a peroxisomal membrane component selected as a parameter also shows non-linear characteristics (Figure 13.5) (Groß, 1994).

It must be pointed out, however, that the results of the above-mentioned in vivo studies could not provide conclusive evidence for the presence of non-linearity and for its causes. The reasons for this are the following:

- The relatively great individual variability with in vivo experiments.
- The impossibility of establishing a direct causal connection between the application of the active substance and the effect.

However, in vivo studies provide sufficient indications of this connection to justify an additional investigation with other preparations and methods.

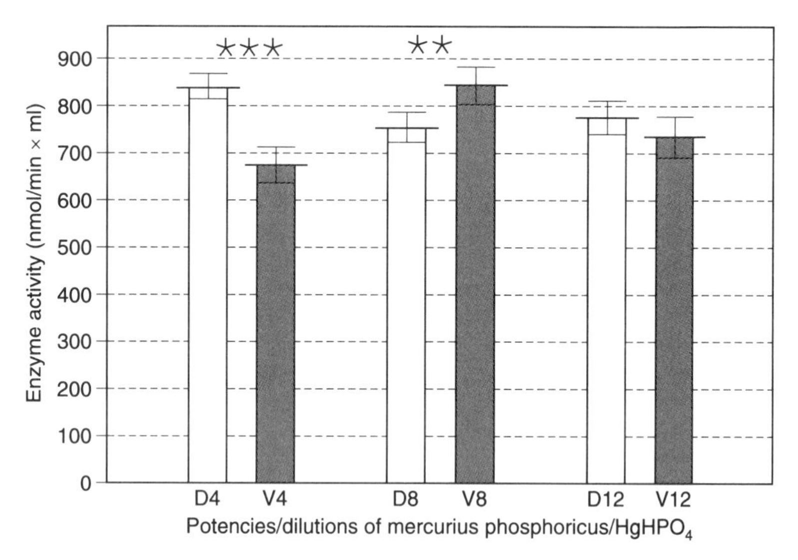

Figure 13.4 Catalytic activity of acid phosphatase. After oral application of mercurius phosphoricus potencies (D4, D8, D12) or $HgHPO_4$ dilutions (10^{-4} (V4), 10^{-8} (V8), 10^{-12} (V12) over a period of seven days, the rats (male Charles River Wistar rats) were decapitated and their livers removed. Activity of acid phosphatase was determined in crude liver fraction obtained by three successive centriguation steps. Significant differences between potency and corresponding dilution are indicated by asterisks (**: $p < 0.01$; ***: $p < 0.001$).

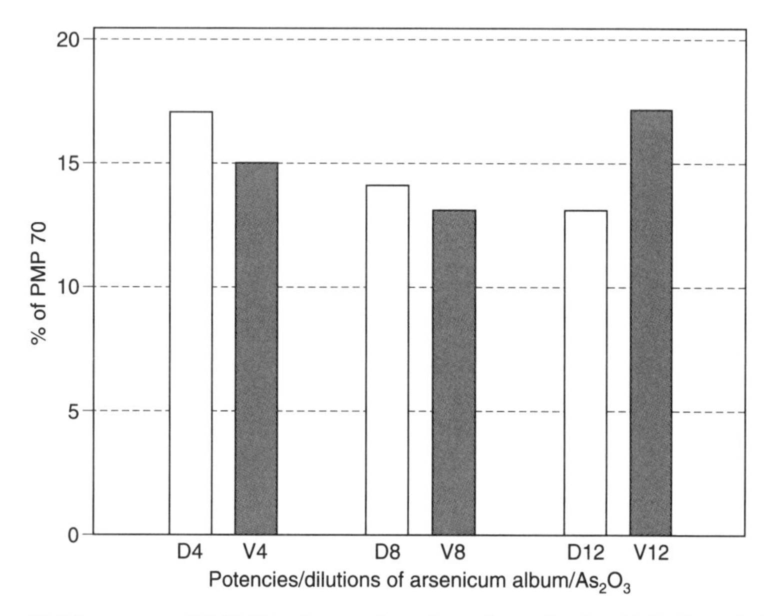

Figure 13.5 Percentage of PMP 70 in the peroxisomal membrane fraction. PMP 70 was isolated from liver peroxisomes of male rats after application of arsenicum album potencies (D4, D8, D12) or As_2O_3 dilutions (10^{-4} (V4), 10^{-8} (V8), 10^{-12} (V12) over a period of seven days.

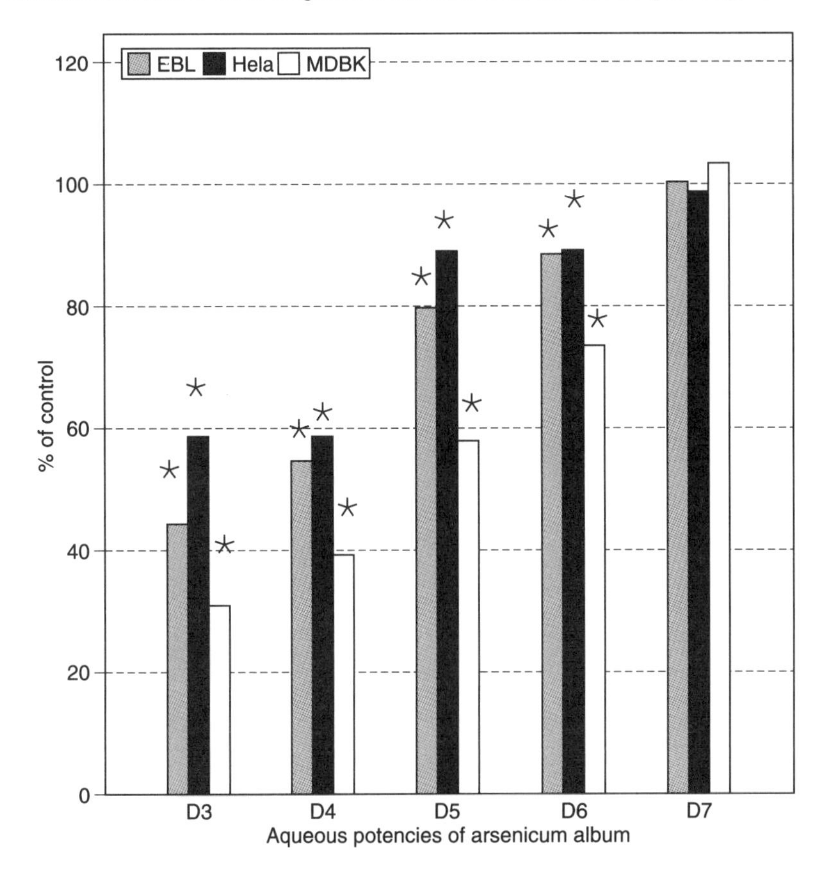

Figure 13.6 Influence of aqueous potencies of arsenicum album on activity of EBL-, HeLa- and MDBK-monolayer cells after incubation of 24h. Values obtained in the absence of arsenicum album were set as 100%. Significant differences between potency and control are indicated by asterisks (*: $p < 0.05$).

Results from in vitro studies

In experiments on **cell cultures** (Then *et al.*, 1996a), it could be established that the intensity of the influence exerted by arsenicum album depends on the type of cell used (Figure 13.6).

The extent of this effect is also influenced by the duration of time cells are exposed to the homoeopathic potencies (Figure 13.7).

Cell-free systems are a particularly valuable tool for studies concerning possible differences in effect between potency and conventional dilution (Dittmann and Harisch, 1996a,b,c; Dittmann, Hentges and Harisch, 1994; Dittmann, Selbach *et al.*, 1994).

Different quantities of the potency D6 of potassium cyanatum exert clearly distinguishable and graded effects on the enzyme, uricase, from hog liver. The conventional potassium cyanide dilution (10^{-6} = V6) with the same concentration behaves similarly. However, the values are on a different level (Figure 13.8).

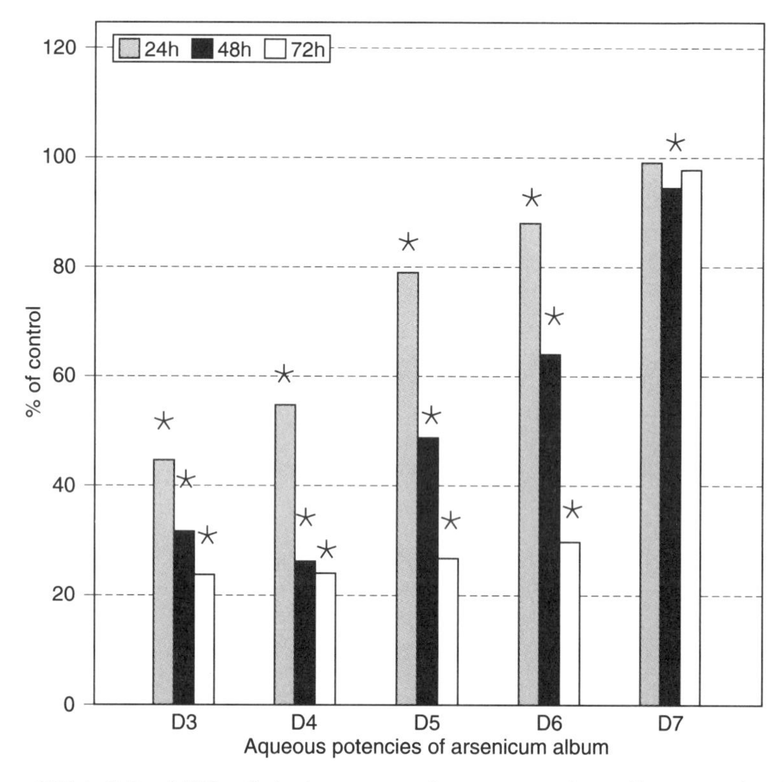

Figure 13.7 Activity of EBL-cells in the presence of aqueous arsenicum album potencies after incubation of 24, 48 and 72h, respectively. Values obtained in the absence of arsenicum album at 24, 48 and 72h were set as 100%. Significant differences between potency and control are indicated by asterisks (*: $p < 0.05$).

The influence exerted on the activity of uricase is accompained by an influence on the enzyme-kinetic parameters like, for example, V_{max}, K_M and the catalytic constant (Figure 13.9).

The microsomal enzyme, cytochrome P-450 2E1-reductase, whose catalytic activity is detected by means of the formation of p-nitrocatechol with HPLC analysis, clearly shows the extent of the effect of ethanol in the cell-free system (Figure 13.10a). For testing in this system, dilutions or potencies should therefore not include an ethanol component. If this is observed, one obtains clearly graded effects with As_2O_3 dilutions (Figure 13.10b).

Not every homoeopathic agent and not every conventional dilution influence every enzyme that is selected as a detection system. Some homoeopathic agents have no effect at all on particular enzymes. Such a case does not imply a general inability to exert an influence. Other active agents can certainly cause effects. In other words, for this type of research, a large number of enzyme systems based on cell-free systems must be available to obtain a picture of the specific effect of a particular homoeopathic agent (Dittmann and Harisch, 1996b).

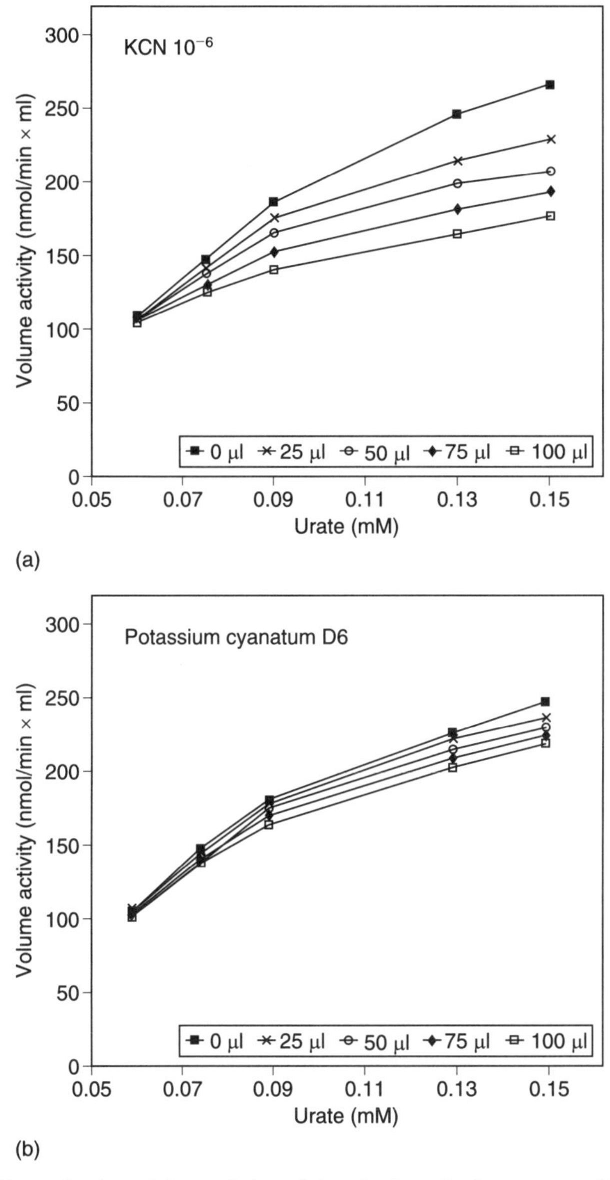

Figure 13.8 Determination of the catalytic activity of uricase in the presence of the indicated substrate concentrations and increasing amounts (25, 50, 75 and 100 µl) of (a) KCN (10^{-6}) or (b) potassium cyanatum (D6).

Integration

Some of the results presented here are not understandable based on the current state of scientific knowledge. This applies especially to the differences in effect between potency and conventional dilution found in the experiments.

However, this non-explainability does not change anything as far as the existence of the data is concerned and it does not make them less reliable.

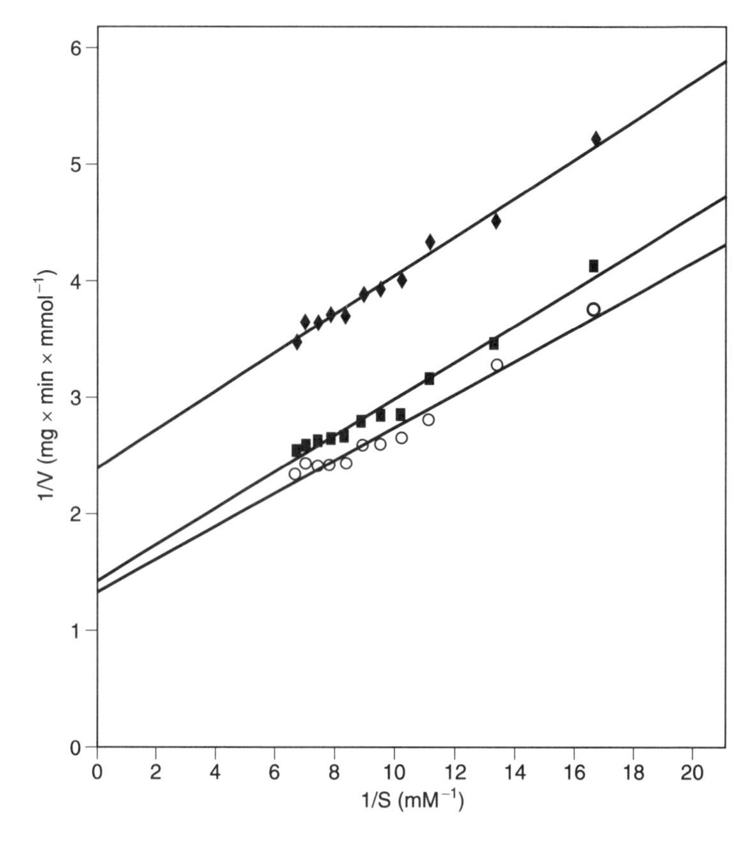

Figure 13.9 Double reciprocal (1/V versus 1/S) Lineweaver-Burk plot obtained by incubation of uricase (from hog liver) in the presence of KCN (dilution 10^{-6}; ◆), potassium cyanatum (potency D6; ■) or in the absence of the agent (o) and increasing concentrations of substrate.
Kinetic data found for uricase in the presence of:

KCN 10^{-6}: V_{max}: 0.421 ± 0.026 [mmol × min^{-1} × mg^{-1}]; K_m: 0.070 ± 0.011 [mM];
potassium cyanatum D6: V_{max}: 0.718 ± 0.070 [mmol × min^{-1} × mg^{-1}]; K_m: 0.114 ± 0.021 [mM];
control: V_{max}: 0.755 ± 0.049 [mmol × min^{-1} × mg^{-1}]; K_m: 0.106 ± 0.010 [mM].

They should arouse scientifically-based and creative curiosity and so stimulate further investigation with other preparations and other methodological approaches.

Comments on high potencies

In the previously discussed views and results presented, no reference is made to the so-called high potencies which are also used in homoeopathy. This does not mean that the methods used here are not suitable tools for high potencies.

The normal scientific way of proceeding when exploring a new subject is not to make the second step before the first. The second step can too easily lead to nothing if the first step does not offer a firm foundation. Only if an

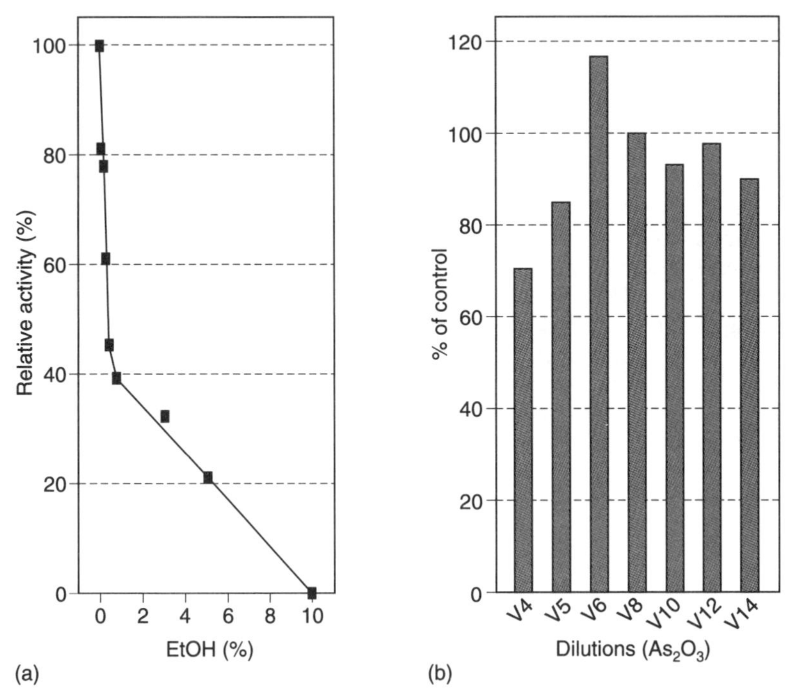

Figure 13.10 Influence of (a) EtOH and (b) As_2O_3 on cytochrom P-450 2E1-reductase. In (a) p-nitrocatechol formation was determined in the presence of solutions containing EtOH as indicated above. In (b) enzyme activity was measured in the presence of As_2O_3 solutions in dilution steps 10^{-4} (V4), 10^{-5} (V5), 10^{-6} (V6), 10^{-8} (V8), 10^{-10} (V10), 10^{-12} (V12) and 10^{-14} (V14). Significant differences between V6 and the other dilution steps used:V6/V10:**; V6/V12:*; in all other cases (including V6/control):***. (*: $p < 0.05$: **: $p < 0.01$; ***: $p < 0.001$.)

adequately precise conception of the effect characteristics of homoeopathic agents in the area of approximately D23 is available – special attention should be paid to non-linearity – can the advance into other areas be promising.

In addition, the previously established effect differences between potencies and conventional dilutions lead only to the conclusion that the process of so-called ‘potentization’ exerts an influence of some sort on the treated substance.

It can be assumed that the type of influence exerted must first be thoroughly investigated before one has the slightest chance of understanding the special characteristics of ‘high potencies’ – provided that they do in fact possess special characteristics. Here too, one can choose other words to express this: only research on the influence of potentization on the substance can provide the methodological tool which is required for working with high potencies.

Until now, the natural sciences have had no cause to attach special importance to the process of the production of potencies which goes beyond the requirements of precision. From this point of view, it is not surprising that until now, no useful model for the possible influences of ‘special potentization’ exists.

Conclusions

Homoeopathic research, or to be more precise, the homoeopathic area of scientific research, is not carried out for the benefit of homoeopathy. It serves exclusively to obtain new knowledge and expand the knowledge horizons of the natural sciences. That the reputation of homoeopathy will be improved in the case of favourable results is a secondary consequence from the scientific point of view.

This integration is imperative and important. For only in this way can it be revealed whether the scientific specialities have not yet investigated a particular field and what the contents of this field are. The importance of this integration is not recognized by most homoeopathic physicians, and its importance is not recognized by most representatives of scientific fields due to the present lack of experimental data.

For both, this non-recognition has negative consequences. A scientist who comes in contact with homoeopathy surely best serves his specific field when he believes it is possible that it is based on the laws of nature. On the other hand, he does little for his field when he regards the lawfulness of homoeopathy as improbable and when he assumes that there is nothing there to investigate.

Genuinely new developments often take place outside of the mainstream of scientific research. Career-related anxieties, combined with the difficulty of financing constitutionally guaranteed scientific freedom, act as obstacles to new developments.

This has a great deal to do with the so-called change in paradigms which many, mostly on the homoeopathic side, regard as overdue. However, it obeys no magical formula: one must work hard to achieve it.

To do this, facts and not words are needed. From this point of view, homoeopathy is not madness, but a real challenge for science. One should not miss this favourable opportunity to discover something new.

References

Dittmann, J. and Harisch, G. (1993) Einfluß potenzierter Substanzen auf Enzyme aus verschiedenen Kompartimenten der Rattenleber. *Dt. J. f. Hom.*, **12**, 291–300.

Dittmann, J. and Harisch, G. (1994) Temperature dependent influence of As_2O_3, $HgHPO_4$ and KCl on lysosomal acid phosphatase isolated from rat liver. *Biochem. Mol. Biol. Internat.*, **34**, 361–5.

Dittmann, J. and Harisch, G. (1995) An automated microtitre plate assay for acid phosphatase as a model system for studying the influence of small amounts of Hg^{2+}-ions on enzyme activity. *Med. Sc. Res*, **23**, 127–9.

Dittmann, J. and Harisch, G. (1996a) Etablierung eines Modellsystems zur Detektierung unterschiedlicher Wirkungen von Potenz und konzentrationsgleicher Verdünnung dargestellt am Beispiel der Uricase aus Schweineleber. *Forsch. Komplementärmed.*, **3**, 64–70.

Dittmann, J. and Harisch, G. (1996b) Zytosolische Glutathion-S-Transferasen und Xanthin-Oxidase/-Dehydrogenase als Indikatoren für die unterschiedliche Wirkung von Potenz und konzentrationsgleicher Verdünnung. *Forsch. Komplementärmed.*, **3**, 176–83.

Dittmann, J. and Harisch, G. (1996c) Characterization of differing effects caused by homeopathically prepared and conventional dilutions using cytochrome P450 2E1 and other enzymes as detection systems. *J. Alternat. Compl. Med.*, **2**, 279–90.

Dittmann, J., Hentges, A. and Harisch, G. (1994) Homoeopathic potencies and equally concentrated conventional dilutions as inhibitors or stimulators of acid phosphatase from potato. *Pharm. Pharmacol. Lett.*, **4**, 40–3.

Dittmann, J., Selbach, A.-C., Hentges, A. and Harisch, G. (1994) Use of urate oxidase as a test system to characterize the effect of homoeopathic potencies and of equally concentrated conventional dilutions. *Pharm. Pharmacol. Lett.*, **4**, 19–22.

Groß, M. (1994) Wirkungen konventioneller Verdünnungen und homöopathischer Potenzen der jeweils gleichen Ausgangsstoffe auf Enzymaktivitäten und die Membranstruktur von Peroxisomen der Rattenleber. Inaugural dissertation, Tierärztliche Hochschule, Hannover.

Harisch, G. and Kretschmer, M. (1990) Jenseits vom Milligramm. Springer Verlag, Berlin.

Harisch, G., Kretschmer, M. and Riemann-Gürlich, C.E. (1992a) Effekte kleinster Wirkstoffmengen – ein Beitrag zur Homöopathieforschung. *Dt. Tierärztl. Wschr.*, **99**, 343–5.

Harisch, G., Kretschmer, M. and Riemann-Gürlich, C.E. (1992b) Der D8-Effekt: Eine Herausforderung für die Homöopathieforschung. *Therapeutikon*, **9**, 386–92.

Hentges, A. (1994) Mineralische Homöopathika und konzentrationsgleiche konventionelle Verdünnungen: Wirkungsunterschiede auf subzellulärer Ebene. Inaugural dissertation, Tierärztliche Hochschule, Hannover.

Kretschmer, M. and Harisch, G. (1992) Lysosomen und Peroxisomen als Zielorganellen für einen Nachweis der Wirkung ausgewählter Homöopathika. *Internist. Praxis*, **32**, 177–81.

Theenhaus, U., Dittmann, J. and Harisch, G. (1993) Unterschiedliche Wirkungen von homöopathischen Potenzen und konventionellen Verdünnungen auf spezifische Leberenzyme der Ratte – ein *in vivo* Versuch. *Dtsch. Tierärztl. Wschr.*, **100**, 485–7.

Theenhaus, U., Dittmann, J. and Harisch, G. (1995) Potenz und Verdünnung, gleiche Konzentration – unterschiedliche Wirkung? *AHZ*, **240**, 151–6.

Then, C., Dittmann, J., Schütte, A., Bauer, J. and Harisch, G. (1996a) In vitro-Untersuchungen zur Wirkung von Arsenicum album Potenzen an Zellkulturen mit Hilfe des MTT-Testes. *Forsch. Komplementärmed.*, **3**, 222–8.

Then, C., Dittmann, J., Schütte, A., Bauer, J. and Harisch, G. (1996b) In vitro-Untersuchungen zur Wirkung homöopathischer Potenzen von Thuja occidentalis an Zellkulturen mit Hilfe des MTT-Testes. *Forsch. Komplementärmed.*, **3**, 280–7.

Chapter 14

Homoeopathy and the mammalian cell: programmed cell recovery and new therapeutic strategies

Roeland van Wijk and Fred A.C. Wiegant

Introduction

The essence of homoeopathy is stimulation of self-recovery by application of the similia principle. Two questions are at issue here: 'What do we know about the regulatory principles underlying recovery that are targeted in homoeopathic treatments?' and 'Under what circumstances can these regulatory principles best be investigated?'

Damage and activated recovery mechanisms

There is only a certain image of what self-recovery actually means. It has been noticed that upon damage a mechanism is switched on aimed at withstanding the disturbing condition and at stimulating recovery. In an organism, the regulation of this self-recovery does seem to take place at more than one level. In general, organs are functionally disordered or damaged because they contain low-functioning or dead cells. Regaining normal functioning depends on the ability of the cells to recover and replace the dead or dying cells. In fact, organ damage is a result of an imbalance between the stimulation of the recovery mechanism and the deleterious consequences of the disturbing condition. It thus is prevented when the recovery and protective capacity exceeds the further infliction of injury.

At cellular level it is then useful to determine what actually happens to a cell in a life-threatening situation. The fact that normal recovery processes work optimally most of the time (e.g. during normal wound healing) indicates that the cell contains regulatory systems which can be described as 'self-recovery'. In case of disorder recovery mechanisms are switched on, leading to prevention of further infliction of injury at the cellular level and to a temporal promotion of cell proliferation. If in such a case the molecular damage is so serious that repair is inadequate and proliferation is no longer stimulated the appropriate organ is on the verge of collapse.

For homoeopathic research it is of major importance to examine how a damaged and thus disordered cell can stay alive and to understand how to adjust or stimulate this self-recovery.

A central aspect of toxicity lies at the level of proteins and is termed 'proteotoxicity'. When cells have been exposed to toxic substances, such as cadmium or arsenite, the structure of many proteins changes. This interferes with the internal interactions of the constituent amino acids so that the right structure can no longer be maintained, leading to functional inactivation of protein molecules. There is also a risk that these now abnormal protein molecules are capable of complexing with other structures in the cell. To sum up, the development of abnormal protein complexes seems to be an important event leading to disordered cellular physiological processes, and is therefore the basis of loss of functionality, cellular damage and cell death.

To understand self-recovery it is important to know the mechanisms that are activated when damage occurs to the proteins and to learn how a cell copes with these damaged life-threatening molecules. In other words, how it recovers from such damage and in what way it develops resistance to a repeat performance. The cellular recovery mechanism involves a number of highly specialized proteins that recognize reactive parts of abnormal proteins.

These proteins are named in different ways. They are more commonly named after the cause of their stimulation, such as 'heat shock proteins' (due to the observation that they are strongly induced upon exposure to enhanced temperature), or 'stress proteins' (since they appear to be induced not only by a heat shock, but by a large variety of cellular stressors). However, they are also named after their function, such as 'chaperone proteins' (since they form complexes with proteinaceous and other cellular structures in order to prevent premature or deleterious interactions between proteins) or 'protector proteins' due to their essential function in the process of programmed cell recovery. In this respect, the protector proteins play a crucial role in reshaping of the damaged proteins into functional units and are thus responsible for development of resistance against damaging conditions. There are a range of different protector proteins. This makes the study of the regulation of self-recovery more complicated but it does lead to a highly versatile molecular system.

The quantity of protector proteins available in the cell decreases under adverse conditions. As long as the essential protector proteins are available in a cell, damage is reduced to a minimum. However, when a shortage arises, as in the case of damage, it will then of course be necessary to step up the production of these protector proteins. Only by increase of this production in a drastic way may the cell prevent its death.

The replenishment of these protector proteins starts with activation of the protector-protein gene promoters on DNA by binding of specific DNA-binding factors, called heat shock transcription factors (HSFs), on their appropriate DNA sites. The binding to a promoter constitutes a signal that triggers transfer of information from DNA into mRNA, eventually leading to new protector proteins. Whether or not a DNA-binding factor binds to its DNA depends on the quantitive level of protector proteins in a cell. The genome is only specifically activated to trigger synthesis of additional protector proteins when their synthesis is invoked. Normally, a specific protector protein species, hsp70, and this DNA-binding factor, HSF, form a complex which provides the basis for regulation of mRNA induction. When protector proteins are required to neutralize abnormal proteins this complex dissociates, causing release of HSF which then interacts with a promoter and thus induces mRNA production. This sets off the process of synthesis of new protector proteins. When more than sufficient new protector proteins have been produced the specific species will again complex with HSF, leading to its abstraction from the DNA, thus ending mRNA production. In terms of systems theories, one might say that this is the autoregulation loop which forms the basis of the damage-induced recovery process.

To sum up, the integrity of the cell system depends not only on the available protective proteins but also on the speed of activation of the mechanism. In turn this is considered to be a major determinant of the recovery process, and thus the duration and severity of the disturbed state.

Recovery is stimulated by application of low doses of damaging conditions

According to homoeopathic vision, recovery may be stimulated by all kinds of substances provided that they are applied in a specific way. Of all substances the one chosen for stimulation of recovery is the one capable of producing the situation of disorder resembling most closely the disordered state. In other words, what matters is the resemblance between symptoms of a disturbed system and symptoms caused by an applied substance in a healthy system. This has been defined as the similia principle. For the cell biologist it is important to concentrate on the most elementary level where the changes in symptoms manifest themselves. In view of this, the similia principle can be tested at the cellular level in its most elementary form by determining the extent to which recovery is stimulated by a small dose of the same substance which, in the first instance, was responsible for upsetting the system or making it 'ill'. The following expectations are formulated with regard to testing the similia principle on the cellular level.

The process of recovery and building up of protection will be stimulated with a smaller dose of the substance needed to disturb the system. This stimulation will show itself in increased synthesis of protector proteins and increased resistance to the disturbing agent. For instance, when arsenite is applied as a disturbing agent, recovery will be stimulated by application of a small dose of arsenite and not, or to a lesser extent, by (non)-related agents such as temperature shocks or small doses of cadmium.

This hypothesis has been studied using three different stressor conditions: a temperature shock followed by mild fever-like temperatures, a damage-inducing treatment with arsenite or cadmium followed by low doses of arsenite or cadmium, respectively. Then, the effects of cross-application of these stressor conditions were studied in order to evaluate the specificity of the similia principle.

Heat-shocked cells

Directly following an acute high-temperature heat treatment cells are thermosensitive and thus exhibit an increased sensitivity to further hyperthermic temperatures of 38–42°C. This is commonly evaluated by a step-down heating protocol in which the initial heat treatment is immediately followed by a second treatment at a lower hyperthermic temperature (Schamhart *et al.*, 1992). In the first studies on the influences of these step-down thermal conditions an enhanced synthesis of protector proteins could be demonstrated in Reuber H35 rat hepatoma cells, the cell line used in our studies (Schamhart *et al.*, 1992). In further studies it was then determined whether the increase of heat shock mRNA after heat stress was also thermosensitized. To this end the induction of mRNAs for hsp68 and hsp84 after application of step-down heating was studied. Step-down heating was initialized by a pretreatment of 30 minutes at 41.5, 42.5 or 43.5°C, followed by continuous incubation of the cells at a lower hyperthermic temperature (40 or 41°C). After a mild pretreatment (41.5°C), the mRNA level of hsp68 in the cells did increase in subsequent incubations at 40°C, although continuous incubation at 40°C alone did not exhibit this effect. This increase was even more pronounced at the secondary temperature of 41°C. Interestingly, an enhanced occurrence of thermotolerance was also observed upon applications of mild step-down heatings. In contrast, cell cultures treated with a severe heat shock showed an inhibited or delayed synthesis of hsp mRNA when post-treated at 40 or 41°C. Under these conditions the development of thermotolerance did not take place either. These data imply that a shift in sensitivity occurs depending on the severity of the pretreatment temperature of the step-down heating protocol (Van Wijk *et al.*, 1994).

Arsenite-shocked cells

With respect to the regulation of cellular sensitivity to stressors other than heat, the phenomenon of an arsenite-induced sensitization towards arsenite has recently been demonstrated (Wiegant *et al.*, 1993). Previously, arsenite had been shown to be an effective inducer of various protector proteins in a variety of mammalian cells.

With respect to recovery, studies were then aimed at determining whether the induction of protector protein synthesis, their mRNAs and the development of tolerance after arsenite application had been sensitized to low concentrations of arsenite. Using a step-down treatment, consisting of a 1-hour pretreatment with 100 or 300 μM arsenite followed by an incubation with a lower concentration (1–10 μM), H35 cells were shown to exhibit increased sensitivity to low concentrations of sodium arsenite with respect to induction of protector proteins and tolerance development. It was observed that under conditions of enhanced sensitivity an additional increase occurred in the synthesis of protector protein mRNAs, as exemplified by hsp68 mRNA behaviour, as well as in their respective products when low concentrations of arsenite were applied to arsenite pretreated cells. Since effects of these low concentrations could not be observed in non-pretreated cells, the effect of step-down treatments thus results in higher effects than can be expected based on summation of the two treatments. Furthermore, we observed that under arsenite step-down conditions, the development of tolerance was enhanced compared with the level of tolerance obtained by a single treatment with either 100 or 300 μM arsenite for 1 hour in cells further untreated with low concentrations of the original stressor (Ovelgönne *et al.*, 1995b).

The concentration of the secondary treatment which leads to a maximal stimulation of the development of tolerance is dependent on the concentration of the pretreatment. When a relatively high concentration of arsenite was used in a pretreatment, the subsequent application of 1 μM did lead to a maximal enhancement of tolerance whereas development of tolerance was inhibited following 10 μM. In contrast, cells pretreated with a relatively low concentration of arsenite demonstrated a maximal enhancement of tolerance following 10 μM. The results thus are comparable to our previous results on step-down heating conditions, where a difference was observed between mild and severe step-down conditions (Van Wijk *et al.*, 1994).

Cadmium-shocked cells

The aim of this third series of studies was to test the hypothesis that a cadmium-induced cellular stress response can be modulated by a subsequent application of low concentrations of the same ion. It was shown that exposure of H35 cells to cadmium concentrations of 10 or 30 μM for 1 hour leads to an initial sensitization towards a secondary treatment with cadmium. Furthermore, incubations for 1 hour in the presence of 10 μM of cadmium do again induce the synthesis of the major protector proteins except now for hsp60. A step-down cadmium regime, i.e. a pretreatment of 1 hour with 10 or 30 μM immediately followed by incubations with lower concentrations of cadmium (ranging from 0.03 to 1 μM), leads to additional increases in protector protein synthesis. No effect of these low concentrations on synthesis of protector proteins could be observed in non-pretreated cells. The sensitized cells also develop a higher level of tolerance in the presence of the above-mentioned low concentrations of cadmium (Wiegant *et al.*, 1997).

In summary, from the results of various experiments it can now be concluded that during a period of enhanced sensitivity, low concentrations of the original stressor enhance synthesis of protector proteins and do induce higher levels of tolerance in comparison with cells which only received a primary stressor treatment.

Now, the question of specificity remains: whether the degree of stimulation is related to the similarity between the damage-activated recovery processes induced by different stressor conditions.

Specificity of the low dose effect

With respect to the specificity of this recovery-enhancing effect of low doses, we determined whether hsp-induction in sensitized cells can also be stimulated by low doses of other (non)-related stressors. The specificity of the similia principle will then reveal itself by the extent to which self-recovery is stimulated by the degree of relatedness between the primary effect of the disturbing compound and the secondary effect of the different substances which are applied to a system.

Studies were again performed with Reuber H35 rat hepatoma cells but now with a cadmium-resistant variant line. A number of experiments were performed in which pretreatments were either given as a heat shock (30 minutes 41.5°C), with sodium arsenite (100 μM for 1 hour) or with cadmium chloride (100 μM for 1 hour). When the induced patterns of protector proteins were compared between heat shock and arsenite, a higher degree of similarity (77.2%) was observed in comparison with the induced patterns of these proteins by heat shock and cadmium (53.8%). The similarity of induction patterns by arsenite and cadmium (64.0%) ranked intermediate.

After the pretreatments the cultures were then exposed to low conditions of either heat (40 or 40.5°C), arsenite (3 or 10 μM), or cadmium (3 or 10 μM) as opposed to incubations at control conditions (37°C). The stimulating effect on the synthesis of various protector proteins was then studied. The application of heat shock, arsenite or cadmium at subliminal conditions to damaged cells early in their recovery yielded a different degree of stimulation of protector protein synthesis, as could be expected because of the different degree of similarity of these stressors. In this respect, application of low doses of arsenite to heat-shocked cultures showed a larger stimulation of hsp synthesis in comparison with the application of a low dose of cadmium to heat-shocked cultures (Van Wijk and Wiegant, 1994). Further studies applying detailed quantitative analysis of the hsp patterns will be presented elsewhere.

In summary, the degree of similarity in the induced pattern of protector proteins by the disturbing conditions applied in high and low dose is reflected in the degree of extra synthesis of protector proteins upon low dose application. These observations confirm the specificity of the low dose effect.

Specific desensitization

A particular aspect of stressors is, that as part of the recovery process, the cells show a biphasic change in their sensitivity towards this stressor. An initially enhanced sensitivity (sensitization) towards a second application of the same stressor is followed by a reduced sensitivity (desensitization or tolerance) at a later time. According to previous definitions, 'tolerance' is described as a stressor-induced cellular resistance towards a stress treatment, whereas 'sensitization' is defined as an increase in cellular susceptibility for a stress treatment. The biphasic change in sensitivity was observed after heat treatments, after treatments with arsenite (Wiegant *et al.*, 1993) or after treatments with cadmium (Wiegant *et al.*, 1997). The changes in sensitivity are usually monitored in terms of survival, but it also carries consequences for the stressor-induced synthesis of protector proteins. In this respect, it has been observed that during and after the period of heat-induced increased synthesis of protector proteins, a state of refractoriness (or tolerance) exists with respect to further induction of the synthesis of protector proteins by a second heat shock (Tuijl *et al.*, 1993). This phenomenon of a temporal state of tolerance has also been studied using fractionated arsenite treatments. Thus, it has been shown that exposure of H35 cells to a sodium arsenite step-down protocol leads to increased sensitivity to low concentrations of sodium arsenite shortly following exposure to the high concentration, but not when the low concentration was applied 4 hours after the pretreatment (Ovelgönne *et al.*, 1995b). These observations led to the conclusion that the capacity to stimulate recovery by an identical substance is a transient phenomenon. The question now to be raised is whether specific non-identical conditions are able to stimulate recovery for longer periods of time.

In a number of earlier studies the effects of two or more stressors were compared and stressor-specific patterns of induced hsps have been described for various eukaryotes. In general, these studies favour the idea that different sets of proteins are induced by different stressors. For Reuber H35 rat hepatoma cells, comparisons of stressor-induced protector molecules under conditions of similar impact on cellular physiology have supported this idea that different patterns of protector proteins are induced by different stressors (Wiegant *et al.*, 1994; Ovelgönne *et al.*, 1995).

The specificity of desensitization of protector protein re-induction was tested employing the three previously mentioned stressors (heat shock, sodium arsenite and cadmium chloride) as primary and secondary inducers of protector proteins (Wiegant *et al.*, 1996). With respect to the existence of stressor-specific patterns of protector protein induction and the stressor specificity in the refractory period, it is concluded that the pattern of protector proteins induced by a secondary applied stressor shows a stressor specificity which seems to be independent of any pretreatment. The pattern of protector protein re-induction is not influenced by the type of stressor used in the pretreatment. However, the primary stressor strongly influences the degree of re-induction of this full pattern of protector proteins with a high degree of specificity. Thus, re-induction following cadmium as the secondary stressor is most severely inhibited in cadmium-pretreated cells, while re-inductions following arsenite and heat shock are specifically inhibited in arsenite- and heat shock-pretreated cells respectively.

From the data obtained it is concluded that a more common denominator does apparently regulate the coordinate expression of a group of protector proteins.

Discussion

The possible implication of the results mentioned so far is that increased production of stress-specific protector proteins and development of tolerance can be obtained in long term incubations with application of a stressor which induces a similar pattern of protector proteins as the primary stressor without being identical to this primary stressor. A stimulatory effect by application of an identical compound can only be observed in the early stages of recovery.

As the pattern of protector protein synthesis is an expression of the molecular programme of recovery, the specificity of the similia principle in the stimulation of recovery does reveal itself in the degree of relatedness between the effects of the disturbing compound on protector proteins and the extent to which this pattern of protector proteins is stimulated by low doses of a compound offered to a disturbed system.

Conclusion

The studies on the similia principle at the cellular level are without doubt significant for our understanding of a new approach in stimulation of programmed recovery processes at the cellular level. The role of cellular recovery processes for an organ's functionality has been discussed at the beginning of this article. Therefore it is to be expected that the application of low doses according to the similia principle offers exciting opportunities for developing new avenues of therapeutic intervention.

Acknowledgement

Dr C.A. van der Mast is gratefully acknowledged for critical reading of the manuscript. This work has been supported by the HomInt organization.

References

Ovelgönne, J.H., Bitorina, M. and Van Wijk, R. (1995a) Stressor-specific activation of heat shock genes in H35 rat hepatoma cells. *Toxicol. Appl. Pharmacol.*, **135**, 100–109.

Ovelgönne, J.H., Wiegant, F.A.C., Souren, J.E.M., Van Rijn, J. and Van Wijk, R. (1995b) Enhancement of the stress response by low concentrations of arsenite in arsenite-pretreated H35 hepatoma cells. *Toxicol. Appl. Pharmacol.*, **132**, 146–55.

Schamhart, D.H.J., Zoutewelle, G., van Aken, H. and Van Wijk, R. (1992) Effects on the expression of heat shock proteins by step-down heating and hypothermia in rat hepatoma cells with a different degree of heat sensitivity. *Int. J. Hyperthermia,* **8**, 701–16.

Tuijl, M.J.M., Cluistra, S., van der Kruijssen, C.M.M. and Van Wijk, R. (1993) Heat-induced unresponsiveness of heat shock gene expression is regulated at the transcriptional level. *Int. J. Hyperthermia*, **9**, 125–36.

Van Wijk, R., Ovelgönne, J.H., de Koning, E., Jaarsveld, K., Van Rijn, J. and Wiegant, F.A.C. (1994) Mild step-down heating causes increased transcription levels of hsp68 and hsp84 mRNA and enhances thermotolerance development in Reuber H35 hepatoma cells. *Int. J. Hyperthermia*, 10, 115–25.

Van Wijk, R. and Wiegant, F.A.C. (1994) Cultured mammalian cells in homeopathy research; the similia principle in self-recovery. Utrecht, Utrecht University, 1–230.

Wiegant, F.A.C., Souren, J.E.M., Van Rijn, J. and Van Wijk, R. (1993) Arsenite-induced sensitization and self-tolerance of Reuber H35 hepatoma cells. *Cell. Biol. Toxicol.*, **9**, 49–59.

Wiegant, F.A.C., Souren, J.E.M., Van Rijn, J. and Van Wijk, R. (1994) Stressor-specific induction of heat shock proteins in rat hepatoma cells. *Toxicology*, **94**, 143–59.

Wiegant, F.A.C., Spieker, N., Van der Mast, C.A. and Van Wijk, R. (1996) Is heat shock protein re-induction during tolerance related to the stressor-specific induction of heat shock proteins? *J. Cell. Physiol.*, **169**, 364–3.

Wiegant, F.A.C., Van Rijn, J. and Van Wijk, R. (1997) Enhancement of the stress response by minute amounts of cadmium in sensitized Reuber H35 hepatoma cells. *Toxicology*, **116**, 27–37.

Part V

Socioeconomic Aspects

[[BLANK PART-TITLE VERSO]]

Chapter 15

Patients' health beliefs and behaviours

Adrian Furnham

Introduction

Are homoeopathy patients in some sense unique? Are they simultaneously both a fairly uniform group (in terms of beliefs, behaviours, medical history and demography) while being different from patients of orthodox medicine (OM) or other complementary medicine (CM) practices? Are homoeopathy patients drawn to the unique theory and therapy of this speciality or are they mere consumers of different specialities capriciously shopping for health? Are homoeopathy patients more satisfied with, and therefore more loyal to, this practice than those patients of other complementary practitioners?

This chapter will address itself to a number, but not all, of the above questions. Some of the above questions are particularly difficult to answer because of the unavailability of reliable statistics based on large representative samples. Further, the results may well differ from country to country because it is well known that some complementary practices are considerably better accepted and established in some countries than in others.

The focus of this chapter is inevitably on homoeopathy patients and their beliefs. However it will also consider ordinary people's perceptions of homoeopathy.

Homoeopathy was formulated by Dr Samuel Hahnemann who published the first textbook of homoeopathy in 1810. Like herbalists, homoeopaths view the body as being sustained by a vital energy. The task of the homoeopath is also to stimulate this vital force and allow healing to take place. A skilled homoeopath can detect imbalances and dysfunctions before disease actually manifests. Diagnosis takes account of changes that may be physical, sensory, emotional, mental or even moral, and is expressed not in the name of a disease, but in the name of the remedy that corresponds to it. The fundamental principle of treatment is to give a remedy which would provoke an identical symptom complex in the patient on the principle that 'like should be cured by like'. The use of vaccines to stimulate the production of natural antibodies could be seen as a parallel approach. However the aspect of homoeopathy which has caused most controversy is Hahnemann's observation that minute doses were more effective in stimulating healing than conventional doses. Homoeopathic remedies are frequently successively diluted to the point where it seems inconceivable that any single molecule of the original substance could be left. Various explanations are given for this: one is that a dissolved substance leaves an imprint in water after high dilution. Others consider that homoeopathic remedies operate at a subtle level not amenable to scientific investigation. Homoeopathy is used in many minor acute conditions and in a wide range of chronic problems (Fulder, 1984). Furthermore it should be assumed that there are no differences between homoeopathic therapists (Canter and Nanke, 1989).

How do the different complementary therapies differ from each other? What do they have in common? Pietroni (1986) presents a useful classification of the different approaches in complementary medicine. He distinguishes:

- Psychological approaches and self-help exercises such as breathing and relaxation, meditation, exercise regimes and visualization.
- Specific therapeutic methods such as massage, reflexology, aromatherapy and spiritual healing.
- Diagnostic methods, such as iridology, kinesiology and hair analysis.
- Complete systems of healing, such as acupuncture, herbal medicine, osteopathy and chiropractic, homoeopathy and naturopathy.

Despite the many profound differences there are some common themes or similarities across complementary medicine specialities. These include a *vitalistic philosophy* which is the idea that the body, and the psyche (cognitive and emotional) are maintained by an underlying energy or vital force.

Health and disease are a reflection of balance and imbalance within this system, or viewed as an interaction between positive life-enhancing forces and negative destructive forces. Second, the belief in an underlying vital force or energy is closely associated with the view that the body is essentially *self-healing*, and the task of the practitioner is to assist the healing process – a fundamentally gentler approach to treatment than orthodox medicine. Third, complementary therapies tend to have a single, *all-encompassing theory of disease*. Finally, complementary systems of medicine have a view of health that goes beyond the simple absence of symptoms. An ideal state of mental and physical health is implicit in many of the theories.

Although there is no absolute dividing line on clinical, theoretical or professional approaches, there are nevertheless differences of emphasis between orthodox and complementary approaches. Many of these have been discussed, but they are helpfully summarized by Aakster (1989) in his comparison of two textbooks, one of orthodox medicine and one edited book on complementary medicine.

While some of Aakster's conclusions are rather extreme and the dimensions too obviously polarized, the different perspectives of orthodox and complementary medicine do emerge. Many of these dimensions are however only likely to be of direct relevance to practitioners, whether orthodox or complementary. The philosophical underpinnings may not be relevant, or even apparent, to many patients. What will matter more to them, and determine whether they attend and later recommend complementary medicine, is whether it appears to help them and the nature of the treatment and the consultation – in other words how the theory and philosophy translate into practice.

In this chapter we will be particularly concerned with homoeopathic patients: their beliefs, attitudes and self-reported behaviours.

Table 15.1 Comparison of orthodox and complementary medicine

Dimension	*Regular, western, orthodox or official medicine*	*Alternative, complementary, integrated medicine*
Model of thinking	'Classical': causality, linearity, specialization, differentiation, materialization, short time perspective	'Perspective': regulation (feedback), interaction, development, connectedness, wholeness, learning
Definition of disease	Organ-specific, accent upon lesion	Functional status, imbalance
Epidemiology	Secondary in interest, fragmentary awareness	General interest in relations to environment
Causation	Linear causality, priority with material factors	Interactive development, material and immaterial factors
Natural history	Accent upon full grown clinical pathology	Interest in (early) development of disease
Pathology	Of central importance	Second in priority
Clinical features	Accent upon organ-bound signs	Interest in complete picture of dysfunctions
Diagnostic procedures	Organ-specific measurement, technical approach, accent upon material	Whole person context, also psychology and energetic, soft methods
Treatment	Organ-specific, technical, accent upon material	Directed at regulation, self-correcting measures also psychology and energetic aspects
Effects	Means-oriented, experimental methods	Goal-oriented, experience based methods
Complications	Secondary in interest, high tolerance for harmfulness	Excluded by choice, low tolerance for harmfulness
Rehabilitation	Secondary in interest, accent upon elimination of disease	Of central importance, orientation upon restoration of health
Care organization	Hospital oriented, differentiated care	Ambulant care, direct access to comprehensive care
Prevention	Secondary in interest, technical and individualized measures	Of central importance, awareness and behaviour of the patient, societal/ environmental measures
Doctor–patient relationship	Secondary in interest, detached concern	Often of prime interest, condition in therapeutic process, education of the patient
Position of patient	Passive, dependent, ignorant	Active, partner, responsible
Cost and burdens	Secondary interest	Certain awareness

Comparative studies

A number of studies have however been undertaken that compare and contrast attitudes, beliefs and self-reported behaviours. All studies in this area face two major methodological problems regarding sampling.

The first is that patients of different therapies often differ from each other not only on their medical problem and history but also on a range of other demographic differences like age, sex, class, etc. Therefore any differences one may find between the different groups may equally be attributed to these differences rather than their health beliefs and behaviours. There are two ways to deal with this. The first is to search out truly comparable groups that are matched on a range of salient variables. The problem with this very expensive strategy is that highly unrepresentative individuals may be over-represented in certain groups because they have to fulfil the profile set in others. The second, probably more reasonable technique is to deal with this issue statistically by 'partialling out' or 'controlling for' these demographic and medical history variables while examining the true differences on the variables that are of primary interest.

The second sampling issue is the problem of generalizability to other regions or countries. It is generally accepted that culture shapes the way patients think about, and maintain their health, and attempt to deal with illness. Thus factors that predict health-related behaviours in one country may be quite different from those that predict in another. Equally it may well be that those factors that statistically reliably discriminate between different patient groups in one country do not do so in another.

Such methodological difficulties are neither insurmountable nor unique but are important for evaluating the research in the area. Alas, various comparative studies in the area have not distinguished between various branches of complementary medical practice and make an analysis of homoeopathic patients impossible (Furnham and Forey, 1994; Furnham and Kirkcaldy, 1996; Furnham and Beard, 1995).

Homoeopathy versus orthodox medicine: patients' beliefs and behaviours

A number of studies have been done each examining a variety of hypotheses concerning the difference between patients of homoeopaths and those of GPs. Though some of the findings have been equivocal without replications others have proved to be fairly robust. It should be pointed out that all the research indicates that the very patients of any CM speciality are exclusively using that speciality. Most CM patients see their CM therapists about specific (often chronic) problems while happily using an OM practitioner for other, particularly acute, illnesses. It would be relatively unusual to find a patient who exclusively uses a homoeopath for *all* their medical consultations. These will be discussed hypothesis by hypothesis.

The mental health of homoeopathic patients

Furnham and Smith (1988) gave two groups of patients a measure of minor psychiatry morbidity. The mean score for subjects visiting the GP was 6.78, while that for subjects visiting the homoeopath 9.17. The difference was statistically significant: ($F = 9.54$, $p < .01$). The results, which are slightly above the norm for both groups (of about 4.0), suggest that the average patient visiting the homoeopath is more psychologically disturbed than the patient visiting the GP. However, if homoeopathic patients have longer illness careers than GP patients and are sicker in the general sense including physical complaints it is perhaps unsurprising that they score highly on measures of psychological illness. Furnham and Bhagrath (1993) confirmed this result. There was a significant difference on the two groups' Langner mental health score, with the orthodox medicine group scoring lower than the homoeopathic group: orthodox patients 23.02; homoeopathic patients 27.11 ($F = 10.08, p < .001$). This does not of course mean that homoeopathic patients are 'mad' but the current data cannot speak to the direction of causality. Whilst it is unlikely that potential psychiatric cases are drawn to homoeopathy, it is much more likely that chronic problems lead (often desperate) people to seek out homoeopathy, and that this leads to an increase in their psychiatric symptomatology.

Resistance to diseases and preventive measures

Do homoeopathy patients have different views about illness prevention? Furnham and Smith (1988) required to two groups to rate the efficacy of eight preventive measures to stay healthy which, it should be pointed out, are measures of intended, not actual behaviour. Only two yielded significant differences between the groups. GP patients thought *regular exercise* was less effective ($F = 7.08, p < 0.01$), but *taking medicines* more effective ($F = 3.93, p < 0.05$) than patients attending a homoeopath.

Subjects were also asked two questions about resistance to illness and disease, one of which yielded significant differences. Homoeopathic patients, more than those visiting a GP, believed their general resistance to illness could be improved ($F = 4.42, p < 0.05$).

Furnham and Bhagrath (1993) found many more differences between the two groups in their study. The nine questions concerning illness prevention showed seven significant differences in the same (to-be-expected) direction. Homoeopathic patients believed more than orthodox medicine patients that a good diet, cutting down on drinking and smoking, reducing stress at work, increasing relaxation time, having a good sleeping pattern and meditation helped prevent illness.

Homoeopathic patients believed in treating the whole person not just the symptoms ($F = 29.13, p < .001$), and also believed more strongly that the body could heal itself than the patients of an orthodox GP ($F = 13.77, p < .01$). Overall, however, there was no difference between the groups in their answer to: 'How satisfied are you with your life?'; 'How resistant would you say you are to illness in general?'; 'Does your lifestyle make you prone to illness?'; and 'Do you believe your general resistance to illness could be improved?' It seems that homoeopathic patients are more interested in health issues. Further, quite naturally they are also more likely to endorse some of the central tenets of homoeopathy concerning the body's ability to heal itself.

Health consciousness

Do homoeopathy patients seek out and pay attention to health information more than orthodox patients? Furnham and Bhagrath (1993) who compared

80 patients from either groups found of the three questions asked, only one yielded a significant result. Homoeopathic patients agreed that they were less likely to take much notice of TV and radio health care recommendations, presumably because they (the advertisements) favoured orthodox medicine. There was no difference between the groups to the questions: 'Do you put a lot of effort into staying healthy?' and 'Do you often read about health care?' This appears to contradict some of the findings from the previous hypotheses, but the limited research addressing the hypothesis obviously requires extension and replication.

Perceived susceptibility to illness

Furnham and Smith (1988) gave their two patient groups 21 medical problems including infections, cardio-vascular problems, neurological and psychosomatic illness, and were asked to rate how likely they were to get them. Various analyses were performed comparing the GP and homoeopath groups, yet *none* reached significance. In other words, there is no difference between the groups in their perceived susceptibility to illness and disease.

Furnham and Bhagrath (1993) had similar findings: only two of the 21 factors yielded a significant result, showing both groups had very similar perceptions of medical risk. However, homoeopathic patients believed themselves more likely to get asthma ($F = 11.24$, $p < .001$) and suffer sleeplessness ($F = 5.92$, $p < .05$) than orthodox medical patients ($F = 6.02$, $p < .05$). Indeed all subjects thought they were fairly unlikely to get all of the illnesses listed. These replicated results seem quite clear: homoeopathy patients do not seek out homoeopaths because (or indeed get educated by them into believing) they are differentially sensitive to different sorts of diseases or illnesses.

Beliefs in the efficacy of treatment

Furnham and Smith (1988) wondered if there are clear differences between OM (GP) and CM (homoeopathy) patients in the way they perceive the efficacy of the treatment given. The six questions on the efficacy of treatment all yielded significant differences. The results showed that both groups believe that medical treatment should concentrate on the 'whole' person, rather than the symptoms, but the homoeopathic group expressed this belief to a far greater degree. The homoeopathic group, more than the GP group, believed that the body can heal itself, which follows their beliefs that their general resistance to illness can be improved. The GP group appear more or less indifferent about leaving their health in the hands of the professionals, but the homoeopathic group come out strongly against this.

This result shows very clearly the disenchantment that CM patients express about regular medicine. But it also shows their relative scepticism with their CM practitioner (see questions 5 and 6). It may well be that many homoeopathic patients are those with chronic problems that they have presented to numerous therapists without a successful cure or release from their suffering. Hence they remain sceptical. This idea contrasts significantly with the OM practitioners who see all patients of CM as gullible, naive people fleeing from science.

Table 15.2 Means and *F* levels for the ANCOVA (analysis of co-variance) between the two groups' response on treatment questions

Questions		*GP*	*Homoeopath*	F *level*
1.	Treatment should concentrate on 'symptoms' rather than on the 'whole' person	3.48	1.95	16.21***
2.	I think my body can help heal itself	4.91	5.57	5.30*
3.	I like to leave my health in the hands of professionals	4.43	2.64	23.25**
4.	How effective do you think the person treating you will be?	5.80	5.21	6.90**
5.	How confident are you that your treatment will end?	5.84	4.98	11.75***
6.	At your last visit to your GP, were you satisfied with your treatment?	6.27	3.70	50.96***

Scale: 1 = strongly disagree; 7 = strongly agree (Q 1, 2, 3, 6).
1 = very; 7 = not at all (Q 4, 5).
***p <0.001; **p <0.01; *p <0.05.

In a related study Furnham and Bhagrath (1993) asked five questions to their two groups about treatment. Homoeopathic patients agreed less than orthodox patients that they liked to leave their health in others' hands, reflecting their scepticism and belief in their personal control over their health. Also, homoeopathic patients expressed less confidence in their treatment and agreed that they were less satisfied on their last visit than orthodox patients, reflecting their scepticism. This certainly suggests that homoeopathic patients are not uninformed optimists when it comes to seeking out homoeopathy, but critical and sceptical clients. Interestingly, homoeopathic patients were more likely to have tried acupuncturist and osteopathic treatment (but not herbalists) than orthodox patients. Under 10 per cent of the orthodox patients had tried complementary practitioners. There was, however, no difference between the groups on the two questions: 'How effective do you believe the person treating you will be?' and 'How confident are you that your treatment will end well?'.

Control over health

Are homoeopathic patients more fatalistic than orthodox medicine patients? The theme of locus of control has been very popular with health education researchers of late. Furnham and Smith (1988) gave GP and homoeopathy patients a question which has four subscales: *self-control over health* (e.g. 'People's ill health results from their own carelessness'); *provider control over health* (e.g. 'Doctors can rarely do very much for people who are sick'); *chance health outcomes* (e.g. 'Recovery from illness has nothing to do with luck'); and *general health threat* (e.g. 'The seriousness of many diseases is overstated').

Only one of the four scales yielded a significant result. Homoeopathic patients had a significantly lower score on the provider subscale. An item-by-item analysis of the items making up the subscale showed that seven of the eight all revealed significant difference in the predicted direction.

Table 15.3 Results from the five questions on treatment preference

Treatment questions (rated on a four-point scale)	*GP* M *(SD)*	*Homoeopath* M *(SD)*	F *ratio*
'I like to leave my health in the hands of the professionals.' (1 = agree, 4 = disagree)	1.98 (0.97)	2.40 (0.96)	10.60**
How effective do you believe the person treating you will be? (1 = very, 4 = not at all)	1.73 (0.58)	1.91 (0.70)	2.79
How confident are you that your treatment will end well? (1 = very, 4 = not at all)	1.82 (0.61)	2.05 (0.77)	4.18
At your last visit to your practitioner, how satisfied were you with your treatment? (1 = very, 4 = not at all)	1.73 (0.70)	2.29 (0.89)	18.79***
Have you ever visited a complementary medical practitioner? (% saying yes)			
e.g. homoeopath	8	92	188.40***
acupuncturist	3	22	13.47***
herbalist	5	13	3.64
osteopath	7	40	27.65***

*p <.05; **p <.01; ***p <.001.

Homoeopathic patients were, by and large, more critical and sceptical about the efficacy of traditional doctors in curing illness. This is very clearly illustrated in the item-by-item analysis of the subscale presented in Table 15.4. However, the difference between groups on the provider control scale is not very surprising in view of the wording of the items which refer to 'doctor' and 'medical' as the provider. Thus if the subjects perceived the homoeopath not to be a doctor (in the conventional sense) the results would simply be a justification of their present course of action. It is relevant that no other subscale showed any difference between the two groups. It may well be that consumers of alternative medicine have long histories of illness and (mal) treatment in the regular sector and have progressed further in their illness career. Hence their disenchantment with traditional medicine.

Furnham and Bhagrath (1993) found a rather different pattern. There were no overall differences on the total subscale scores for chance health outcomes. Similarly, the provider control scale failed to yield a significant difference. The self-control subscale did reveal significant differences (F = 5.15, p <.05) with homoeopathic patients scoring more highly, believing that they were indeed more in control of their health. Four of the seven items showed significant differences, and in all cases GP patients agreed more than homoeopathic patients that: 'There is little one can do to prevent illness' (F = 4.93, p <.05) (reverse scored); 'Healthwise, there isn't much you can do for yourself when you are sick' (F = 5.01, p <.05); and 'Taking care of yourself has little or no relation to whether you get ill' (F = 7.66, p <.05) (reverse scored). Thus, overall the differences were quite consistent. The final scale, general threat to health, did not show an overall difference (F = 0.59, n.s): (F = 6.04, p <.05).

The inconsistency in these findings is important and possibly warrants further research given the great interest of health education in the locus of

Table 15.4 Homoeopath and GP group responses on the four health locus of control subscales
(a) Means and *F* level from the ANCOVA

Subscales		*GP* (N = 44)	*Homoeopath* (N = 43)	F *ratio*
1.	Chance health outcomes	5.01	4.70	1.03
2.	Provider control over health	5.44	4.36	16.93***
3.	Self-control over health	5.14	5.12	0.07
4.	General health threat	3.88	3.67	0.46

Scale: 1 = strongly disagree, 7 = strongly agree

(b) Item-by-item analysis of provider-control scale

		GP	*Homoeopath*	F
1.	Seeing the doctor for regular check-ups is the key factor in staying healthy	4.45	3.32	7.93**
2.	Doctors can rarely do much for sick people	2.36	3.22	4.98*
3.	Doctors relieve or cure only a few problems that their patients have	3.05	4.62	20.33***
4.	Doctors can almost always help their patients feel better	5.29	4.24	10.72**
5.	Recovery from illness requires good medical care more than anything else	5.02	4.34	4.49*
6.	Most people are helped a great deal when they go to the doctor	5.71	4.22	24.13***
7.	Doctors can do very little to prevent illness	3.33	3.46	0.10
8.	Many times doctors don't help their patients get well	2.90	3.88	6.69*

***p <0.001; **p <0.01; *p <0.05

control concept. Many researchers have speculated that patients are drawn to CM because of disenchantment with general practice and the belief that they are in charge of their health. Hence one would expect the significant differences found in the two above studies, but both together in the same study.

Medical history

Furnham and Bhagrath's (1993) study contains eight questions which looked at patients' medical history in terms of their use of treatment. Only four questions showed significant differences but the results are particularly interesting. Homoeopathic patients visited the homoeopath because of a belief in the treatment ($F = 5.28, p < .05$), but more because of dissatisfaction with orthodox medicine ($F = 22.42$, $p < .001$). Yet homoeopathic patients were likely to 'hedge their bets' by staying with orthodox as well as a complementary medicine ($F = 28.71$, $p < .01$). It is well known that many complementary medicine practitioners also use orthodox medicine for specific problems beyond the scope of the particular complementary therapy. Interestingly, homoeopathic patients expected to live longer than orthodox patients ($F = 6.36$, $p < .05$).

This area of research has been woefully neglected, partly because of the difficulty of getting a good medical history by questionnaires or by non-medically trained researchers. Indeed it is by obtaining the medical history and 'career' of patients that we may more fully understand their motives for seeking out, and staying with, CM practitioners.

Overall these studies have shown homoeopathy patients more sceptical to orthodox medicine; more interested in their own health and believing they can do something about it; and with higher psychiatric morbidity. There is much less evidence that homoeopathy patients have different or unusual views about the cause of illness or are anti-scientific.

Comparing homoeopathy with other CM groups

By comparing the beliefs and practices of homoeopathy with say acupuncture and osteopathy patients (as well as patients of conventional orthodox medicine), it may be possible to determine how unique they are. There have been a number of studies that have made these comparisons. Whilst they suffer from the same problems as noted earlier they do allow for the testing of certain hypotheses.

Locus of control

Studies by Furnham, Vincent and Wood (1995) and Vincent, Furnham and Willsmore (1995) both examined health locus of control differences between three different complementary medical groups. Neither study found any evidence of statistical differences, so throwing further doubt at the discriminating nature of health locus of control beliefs between patients of different orthodox or complementary specialities.

Familiarization with therapy

Furnham, Vincent and Wood (1995) asked patients in their four groups (3 CM, 1 OM) to what extent they were familiar with six reasonably well-known complementary therapies by stating whether they had heard about, had tried or would try them. Acupuncture, homoeopathy, and osteopathy patients had of course generally tried their specific therapy unless it was their first appointment when they stated that they would try or had 'heard of' only.

Perhaps the most interesting result from Table 15.5 is the second row ('Have tried'), which shows that patients from all groups admitted to having tried other therapies. This was least evident for chiropractic and naturopathy, but particularly strong for homoeopathy and osteopathy. Thus although the complementary medicine groups were categorized in terms of their current usage, in the past they may have tried other therapies. Again this shows that patients shop for health. Note the enthusiasm homoeopathy patients express for acupuncture and herbalism.

Table 15.5 Familiarization with alternative therapies[a]

Type of treatment	*GP*	*Osteopathy*	*Homoeopathy*	*Acupuncture*
Acupuncture				
Heard about	24	17	18	1
Have tried	4	1	20	53
Would try	21	26	29	1
Chiropractic				
Heard about	16	15	26	24
Have tried	9	8	8	9
Would try	14	22	17	13
Herbalism				
Heard about	28	17	15	11
Have tried	4	1	11	13
Would try	17	20	32	27
Homoeopathy				
Heard about	25	12	1	10
Have tried	5	21	62	30
Would try	18	19	7	12
Naturopathy				
Heard about	16	11	18	15
Have tried	1	3	8	8
Would try	3	11	17	9
Osteopathy				
Heard about	28	2	19	7
Have tried	7	53	18	32
Would try	16	3	19	3

[a] Missing subjects indicated that they had not heard of the therapy in question; for example, over half of the subjects had not heard of naturopathy.

Scientific health beliefs

Is the homoeopathy patient simply fleeing from science? Have they lost faith in medical science? Furnham, Vincent and Wood (1995) asked their three CM patients and one OM (GP) group 16 questions, e.g.: 'When it comes to medical treatment, patients should always follow their doctor's advice'; 'We are fortunate to live in a world of medical excellence – skilled surgery, highly trained professional care, etc.'; 'Modern therapeutic achievements (e.g. liver heart transplants) are important contributions to progress in health care'; 'If I were ever seriously ill, I would have a lot of faith in doctors to find a cure'; 'Medicine is a science and should be based on rigorous scientific principles'.

These made up four factors (the above were all from the first factor) and the groups were then compared (Table 15.6).

- **Factor 1. Faith in medical science.** Significant difference found between groups, with the GP group showing most faith while the acupuncture group showed the least: significantly less than any of the other three groups.
- **Factor 2. Importance of a 'healthy mind.'** Significant difference found between groups, with acupuncture patients placing the most importance on a healthy state of mind, significantly more so than either homoeopath patients or GP patients, who place the least importance on state of mind.

Table 15.6 Results of ANCOVA on scientific health belief factors

Factor		*GP*	*Ost*	*Hom*	*Acu*	F *ratio*
1.	Faith in medical science	5.32	5.03	4.85	4.14	4.16***
2.	Importance of 'healthy mind'	5.88	6.22	5.99	6.47	5.34***
3.	Harmful effects of medical science	4.49	4.80	4.96	5.40	4.38***
4.	Scientific methodology	4.39	4.36	4.29	3.49	5.92***

The higher the score the more they agree with that factor. ***p <0.001

Table 15.7 Health beliefs of complementary and general practice patients with ANCOVA results

	Acupuncture	*Homoeopathy*	*Osteopathy*	*GP*	F *ratio*/P *ANCOVA*
Scientific basis to medicine	3.46[a]	4.15[b]	4.20[b]	4.74[b]	$F = 6.15$***
Psychological factors in illness	6.34	6.21	6.01	5.85	$F = 0.25$
Harmful effects of medicine	5.66[a]	5.29[b]	4.69[b]	4.45	$F = 2.72$*

Means with similar superscripts are not significantly different. ***p <.001; *p <.01.

- **Factor 3. Harmful effects of medical science.** Significant difference found between groups. The GP group was least concerned, with the acupuncture group most concerned, significantly more than the GP group.
- **Factor 4. Scientific methodology.** Significant differences were found between groups. The GP group showed most support for this while the acupuncture group showed least support, significantly less than any of the other three groups.

In a similar study Vincent, Furnham and Willsmore (1995) looked at various health beliefs, particularly relating to the scientific status. The results (Table 15.7) show some interesting differences.

The acupuncture group attached significantly less importance to science than the GP group and were more worried about the harmful effects of medicine than either the GP or osteopathic group. The homoeopathic group, although attending a NHS hospital, were also more concerned about the harmful effects of medicine than the GP group. Precisely why acupuncture patients should be so different from other CM patients is not clear.

Attitudes to GPs

Furnham, Vincent and Wood (1995) found, not surprisingly, interesting differences between various groups' perceptions of therapists. Complementary practitioners were perceived as more sympathetic by all the groups to some extent (i.e. all mean scores past 4 on a 7-point scale), but significant differences were still apparent between groups, with the GP group agreeing least with the statement, while the acupuncture group agreed most significantly more than any of the other three groups.

Table 15.8 Means and *F* levels for patients' 'comparative' perceptions[a]

Items	*GP*	*Osteo-pathy*	*Homoe-opathy*	*Acupunc-ture*	F *ratio*
Compared to GPs, complementary practitioners					
Are more sympathetic	4.41	5.38	5.04	6.31	14.79***
Have more time to listen	4.88	5.54	5.09	6.71	17.50***
Have less knowledge of disease	3.67	3.37	2.83	3.09	2.23
Are more sensitive to emotional issues	4.44	5.32	5.07	6.55	19.28***
Are better at explaining the treatment	4.26	5.49	4.87	5.98	11.47***
Are better at explaining why you are ill	4.26	5.44	4.67	6.15	14.99***

[a] 1 = strongly disagree; 4 = neutral; 7 = strongly agree. ***p <0.001

Again all the groups agreed that complementary practitioners have more time to listen, the GP group agreeing least, while the acupuncture group agreed most; significant differences did exist between the four groups, with the acupuncture group showing significantly stronger agreement than any of the other three. All the groups disagreed with the statement that complementary practitioners have less knowledge of disease (i.e. all group means less than 4), and there were no significant differences between groups, although predictably the GP group showed most support for the statement. All the groups agreed that complementary practitioners are more sensitive to emotional issues, but significant differences did exist between the groups, with the GP group showing least support for the statement, while the acupuncture group showed most support, significantly more than any of the other three groups. The osteopath group showed significantly more agreement with the GP group.

All groups agreed that complementary practitioners are better at explaining treatments. Significant differences did exist, with the GP group showing least agreement, while the acupuncture group showed most, significantly more than either the GP or the homoeopath groups, while the osteopath group showed significantly more support for the statement than the GP group. All groups also agreed that complementary practitioners are better at explaining why a patient is ill. The GP patients showed least agreement, while the acupuncture patients showed most, significantly more than either the GP or homoeopath group, while the osteopath group showed significantly more support for the statement than the GP group.

The perceived efficacy of medicine

Do patients of particular complementary therapies believe them to be particularly effective? On a five-point scale (5 = very effective) Vincent, Furnham and Willsmore (1995) asked acupuncture, homoeopathy, osteopathy and a GP group to rate the efficacy of various specialities. The acupuncture group give significantly higher efficacy ratings than the GP group for acupuncture, homoeopathy and osteopathy. For acupuncture the mean scores are significantly higher than all the other groups, indicating a degree of loyalty to their specific therapy.

Table 15.9 Mean scores for perceived efficacy of complementary therapies with ANCOVA

	Acupuncture	*Homoeopathy*	*Osteopathy*	*GP*	F *ratio*
Acupuncture	3.54	2.52	2.20	2.21	7.28***
Herbalism	3.31	2.81	2.57	2.36	1.48
Homoeopathy	3.07	3.16	2.68	2.05	1.46
Osteopathy	1.81	1.59	1.89	1.60	1.23
Orthodox medicine	2.46	2.89	2.86	2.81	0.952

***$p < .001$

The results of Table 15.9 show two things. First it is only the acupuncturists who have clear self-serving attributes for the efficacy of their own speciality. Second, overall the four groups rate the efficacy of orthodox medicine most highly and osteopathy the least efficient therapy.

Health beliefs and lifestyle

Furnham, Vincent and Wood (1995) asked their three CM and one OM groups 20 questions about their health beliefs and lifestyle which factored into five clear factors.

- **Factor 1 – Satisfaction with GP.** Significant difference found between groups, with the GP group showing the most satisfaction with GPs, while the acupuncture group showed the least, being significantly less satisfied than either the GP group or the homoeopath group.
- **Factor 2 – Healthy lifestyle.** Significant difference found between groups, with acupuncture patients having the most healthy lifestyle significantly more so than either osteopath patients or GP patients, who have the least healthy lifestyle.
- **Factor 3 – Global environmental issues.** Significant difference found between groups. The GP group was least concerned, with the acupuncture group most concerned, significantly more than either the homoeopath or the GP group.
- **Factor 4 – Preventive health measures.** No significant differences were found between groups. Taking the individual questions loading on to this factor, one of the two did reveal significant differences. The question 'Do you often read about health in newspapers, magazines, books, etc.?' is significant, with the acupuncture group being most likely to read about health and the GP group least likely. The question, 'Do you take much notice of health care recommendations from the TV, radio, etc.?' produced no significant differences between groups.
- **Factor 5 – Lack of confidence in prescribed drugs.** Significant differences found between groups, with GP patients showing most confidence while acupuncture patients showed least – significantly less than any of the other three groups.

Overall the acupuncture patients stand out as being most different from the rest.

Table 15.10 Mean item scores and results of ANCOVA on health beliefs and lifestyles

Factor	*GP*	*Osteopathy*	*Homoeopathy*	*Acupuncture*	F *ratio*
Satisfaction with GP	4.85	4.45	4.69	3.84	3.59**
Healthy lifestyle	3.10	3.30	3.68	4.03	2.17*
Global environmental issues	5.74	6.05	5.91	6.51	8.20**
Preventive health measures	3.92	4.32	3.86	4.48	2.29
No confidence in prescribed drugs	1.82	2.01	1.99	2.77	3.78***

***p <0.001; **p <0.01; *p <0.05.

Reason for seeking therapy

Do patients from different CM specialists have different reasons for seeking out treatment by them? Vincent and Furnham (1996) asked over 250 patients from three complementary medicine practices – acupuncture, osteopath and homoeopathy – to complete a questionnaire rating 20 potential reasons for seeking complementary treatment. The reasons that were most strongly endorsed were 'because I value the emphasis on treating the whole person'; 'because I believe complementary therapy will be more effective for my problem than orthodox medicine'; 'because I believe that complementary medicine will enable me to take a more active part in maintaining my health'; and 'because orthodox treatment was not effective for my particular problem'.

Five factors were identified, in order of importance:

1 A positive valuation of complementary treatment.
2 The ineffectiveness of orthodox treatment for their complaint.
3 Concern about the adverse effects of orthodox medicine.
4 Concerns about communication with doctors.
5 The availability of complementary medicine.

Groups were compared, using analysis of co-variance to control for demographic differences between the three patient groups.

Osteopathy patients' reasons indicated they were least concerned about the side-effects of orthodox medicine and most influenced by the availability of osteopathy for their complaints. Homoeopathy patients were most strongly influenced by the ineffectiveness of orthodox medicine for their complaints, a fact which was largely accounted for by the chronicity of their complaints.

Three of the factors showed significant differences between the three patient groups. Acupuncture and homoeopathy patients seemed 'put off' by the potential side-effects of medicine more than the osteopathy group. This was probably due to the nature of the problems they presented with, and possible use of drugs by orthodox doctors. A second difference between the groups indicated that the osteopathy patients rated the availability of their therapy as more important than the other two groups. The final factor, which referred to the ineffective nature of orthodox medicine, was rated most highly by the homoeopathic group, who may have complaints that

Table 15.11 Factor scores by patient group

Factor	*Acupuncture*	*Homoeopathy*	*Osteopathy*	*Mean*	F *ratio/sig*
Value of complementary medicine	3.92	3.88	3.98	3.90	0.11
Poor doctor communication	2.85	2.95	2.89	2.90	0.19
Side-effects of orthodox medicine	3.05_{a}	3.01_{b}	2.67_{ab}	2.91	4.13*
Availability of complementary medicine	2.18_{a}	2.37_{b}	2.91_{ab}	3.66	19.2**
Orthodox medicine ineffective	3.51	3.95	3.52		7.00**

Note: Letters indicate pairs of groups whose means are significantly different ($p < .05$) in Scheffé multiples comparisons. *$p < .01$; **$p < .001$

are particularly resistant to orthodox treatment. This would explain why group differences were no longer found after co-variates, including severity of illness, were controlled for.

Lay people's perceptions of homoeopathy and other therapies

Some studies have looked at how a mixed group of ordinary people have perceived the effectiveness of homoeopathy compared to other complementary specialities as well as orthodox medicine. Vincent and Furnham (1994) gave a questionnaire to 135 British adults of whom 12% had experience of complementary medicine.

This study examined the perceived effectiveness of five different types of alternative medicine (acupuncture, herbalism, homoeopathy, hypnosis and osteopathy) *and* orthodox medicine in treating 25 common complaints ranging from cancer to the common cold. Subjects completed a questionnaire measuring the state of their health; experience of complementary medicine; sources of information about complementary medicine; and perceived effectiveness of orthodox and complementary treatments in the treatment of each condition. Personal accounts of treatment appeared to be particularly important sources of information on complementary medicine, and also highly valued in assessing its effectiveness.

As far as ratings of effectiveness were concerned, they could be effectively classified into four groups:

1 Major medical conditions – appendicitis, bronchitis, cancer, diabetes, heart attack and pneumonia.
2 Minor conditions – common cold, hay fever, insomnia, menstrual problems and migraine.
3 Chronic conditions – allergies, arthritis, asthma, back pain, blood pressure and skin problems.

Table 15.12 Perceived effectiveness by illness type

Type	*Hypnosis*	*Acupuncture*	*Herbalism*	*Homoeo.*	*Osteopathy*	*Orthodox medicine*
Major	1.23	1.41	1.70	1.67	1.24	3.98
Minor	1.95	2.02	2.52	2.23	1.41	3.05
Chronic	1.66	2.26	2.37	2.38	1.92	3.45
Psychological	2.92	2.15	2.02	1.80	1.50	2.48

4 Psychological problems – depression, drinking problems, fatigue, nerves, obesity, stopping smoking, stress and weight loss.

Ratings on these various complaints were arithmetically computed to form four scores per subject. Table 15.12 shows the mean efficacy for each therapy, in each of these four groups of conditions.

Table 15.12 suggests that people were, on the whole, emphatic that orthodox medicine is much more effective in any major illness. Complementary medicine was seen as more effective for minor problems and chronic conditions, though orthodox medicine was still rated as superior. For psychological problems complementary medicine and orthodox medicine were very much equivalent. This suggests that most people are not 'for or against' complementary medicine, but see it as useful in certain specific types of problems – especially those where orthodox medicine is seen as less effective. People are, to some extent, aware that particular complementary therapies should be targeted at particular conditions.

What the results showed was that orthodox medicine was clearly seen, by the great majority of subjects, as being more effective in the treatment of most complaints, especially in the treatment of major, life-threatening conditions. Complementary medicine was seen as more effective in the treatment of minor and chronic conditions, though generally not superior to orthodox medicine. For some specific conditions complementary medicine was seen as the most effective treatment: osteopathy and acupuncture were both perceived as valuable in the treatment of back pain, and herbalism was perceived as a valid treatment for fatigue and stress; hypnosis was seen as useful in the treatment of a variety of psychological problems, and seen as superior to orthodox techniques. The fact that people are able to specify which complementary therapies are likely to be effective in which conditions should make researchers cautious about treating 'complementary medicine' as an umbrella term.

This study has in fact been replicated, this time looking at the perceptions of 82 patients attending a British acupuncture clinic. Vincent and Furnham (1997) asked them to complete a brief questionnaire which covered:

(a) demographic information and experience of complementary medicine;
(b) ratings of the perceived efficacy of acupuncture, osteopathy, homoeopathy, herbalism and orthodox medicine for 16 illnesses, divided into four categories: major, minor, chronic and psychological.

Osteopathy and acupuncture were seen as particularly useful for back pain, with acupuncture being seen as beneficial for other chronic conditions

Table 15.13 Effectiveness of therapies by type of condition

	Acupuncture	*Herbalism*	*Homoeopathy*	*Osteopathy*	*Orthodox medicine*
Chronic	4.00 (0.66)	2.95 (0.87)	2.93 (0.95)	3.18 (0.82)	2.36 (0.89)
Major	2.89 (0.89)	2.45 (0.90)	2.54 (1.00)	1.57 (0.79)	3.61 (0.96)
Minor	3.59 (0.81)	3.38 (0.89)	3.33 (1.08)	1.65 (0.71)	2.23 (1.01)
Psychological	4.12 (0.70)	2.95 (0.97)	2.94 (1.01)	2.15 (0.97)	1.68 (0.72)
Overall	3.66 (0.52)	2.91 (0.75)	2.94 (0.86)	2.14 (0.68)	2.48 (0.71)

Mean and (standard deviation) 1 = not at all effective; 5 = very effective.

Table 15.14 Correlations between attitudes and effectiveness

	Acupuncture	*Herbalism*	*Homoeopathy*	*Osteopathy*	*Orthodox medicine*	*Preference for orthodox medicine*
Harmful effects of medicine	0.05	0.16	0.17	0.13	−0.46***	−0.43***
Importance of psychological factors	0.34***	0.41***	0.31**	0.22	0.16	−0.13
Attitudes to science	0.16	−0.10	−0.08	−0.12	0.54***	0.41**

Correlations ***p <.001; **p <.01

and for psychological problems by these acupuncture patients. Orthodox medicine was seen as least effective at curing chronic and psychological conditions.

Acupuncture patients appear to perceive their own chosen therapy as more effective than other complementary therapies and, for many complaints, as more effective than orthodox medicine. The mean scores (on a 1 to 5 scale) for the effectiveness of major, minor, chronic and psychological conditions, and the mean effectiveness scores for each therapy are shown in Table 15.13. Orthodox medicine is clearly seen, even by complementary patients, as more effective for major, life-threatening conditions but acupuncture is still rated as highly effective even for these complaints.

The 12 attitude questions asked in this study fell into three groups (Table 15.14). They concerned the possible harmful effects of medicine; the importance of psychological factors in the development and maintenance of health and illness; and attitudes to science.

The results substantiate some of the earlier findings. A positive attitude to science was also associated with a strong belief in the effectiveness of orthodox medicine. Further, a belief in psychological factors was associated in the previous study with a belief in the effectiveness of acupuncture and homoeopathy, though once demographic or other attitudinal variables were taken into account these results did not quite reach significance. Significant associations were found however between attitudes to psychological factors and a belief in the effectiveness of herbalism. Associations between perceived effectiveness and the importance of psychological factors in illness do not necessarily mean that patients view complementary therapies as placebos. Patients may be drawn to complementary medicine because it is seen as more able to take a psychological perspective into account. Some complementary therapies (e.g. homoeopathy and some forms of acupuncture) explicitly take emotional factors into account in the diagnoses and underlying theory, though it is not clear how far this matters to (or is indeed noticed by) most patients. It may be that complementary practitioners simply have more time, or are seen to be more receptive to discussing emotional aspects of illness.

The results of this study differ from the previous one in one important respect. In the previous one a stronger, relative belief in orthodox medicine amongst patients of different complementary therapies was associated with attaching less importance to psychological factors in illness. Here in contrast, in a group of people attending a very traditionally oriented acupuncture centre, the distinguishing factors were scientific attitudes and beliefs about harm.

Conclusion

What have these programmatic studies shown us about homoeopathic patients' beliefs? First, homoeopathic patients are different from those exclusively using GPs in orthodox medicine by at least four factors:

- they are more sceptical about and dissatisfied with orthodox medical practice;
- they appear to be more interested in health issues;
- they have a different medical career with associated psychological disturbance; and
- they espouse consistently, but at a fairly rudimentary level, some of the basic tenets of homoeopathy.

Are homoeopathic patients different from those patients who have sought out different forms of complementary medicine? The results of these studies show homoeopathic patients' beliefs and self-reported behaviours to be very similar to those of say osteopathy but somewhat different from acupuncture. There may be various reasons for this. Patients may go to an acupuncturist to relieve quite different symptoms or addictions than they would consider going to a homoeopath. Second, to some extent acupuncture has a vague, somewhat mystical status which may attract quite different types of people.

Yet the results show that CM patients groups are not discrete, and totally loyal to their chosen therapy. Many are interested in, attracted to, and even patients of many different treatments. For some no doubt this is a 'hobby'; others may be pushed by desperation to achieve a cure for a problem. Indeed, it may well be that patients have a fairly sophisticated ideal of health and illness, and what specific problems are best cured by which therapy.

The results of the above studies require replication with different larger cross-cultural samples. There is no reason to believe, however, that many will not be replicated, that is that the above findings will be supported in different patient groups in different countries.

References

Aakster, C. (1989) Assumptions governing approaches to diagnoses and treatment. *Social Science and Medicine*, **29**, 293–300.

Canter, D. and Nanke, L. (1989) Individual variation and symptomatology: A homoeopathic perspective. *British Homoeopathic Research Group Communication*, **19**, 43–91.

Fulder, S. (1984) *The Handbook of Complementary Medicine*. London: Hodder and Stoughton.

Furnham, A. and Beard, R. (1995) Health, just world beliefs and copy style preferences in patients of complementary and orthodox medicine. *Social Science and Medicine*, **40**, 1425–32.

Furnham, A. and Bhagrath, R. (1993) A comparison of health beliefs and behaviours of clients of orthodox and complementary medicine. *British Journal of Clinical Psychology*, **32**, 237–46.

Furnham, A. and Forey, J. (1994) The attitudes, behaviours and beliefs of patients of conventional vs complementary (alternative) medicine. *Journal of Clinical Psychology*, **50**, 458–67.

Furnham, A. and Kirkcaldy, B. (1996) The health beliefs and behaviours of orthodox and complementary medicine clients. *British Journal of Clinical Psychology*, **35**, 49–61.

Furnham, A. and Smith, C. (1988) Choosing complementary medicine: A comparison of beliefs of patients visiting a GP and a homoeopath. *Social Science and Medicine*, **26**, 653–87.

Furnham, A., Vincent, C. and Wood, R. (1995) The health beliefs and behaviours of three groups of complementary medicine and a general practice group of patients. *Journal of Alternative and Complementary Medicine*, **1**, 347–59.

Pietroni, P. (1986) Alternative medicine. *Practitioner*, **23**, 1053–4.

Vincent, C. and Furnham, A. (1994) The perceived efficacy of complementary and orthodox medicine. *Complementary Therapies in Medicine*, **2**, 125–34.

Vincent, C. and Furnham, A. (1996) Why do patients turn to complementary medicine? An empirical study. *British Journal of Clinical Psychology*, **35**, 37–40.

Vincent, C. and Furnham, A. (1997) The perceived efficacy of complementary and orthodox medicine: A replication. *Complementary Therapies in Medicine*, **5**, 85–89.

Vincent, C., Furnham, A. and Willsmore, M. (1995) The perceived efficacy of complementary and orthodox medicine in complementary and general practice patients. *Health Education Research*, **10**, 395–405.

Chapter 16

Economic evaluation of homoeopathy

Adrian R. White

Introduction

Economic evaluation of health care is crucial if a health service is to make the most effective use of resources in the most equitable way. The potential economic benefit of homoeopathy must be considerable in view of the cheapness of the remedies, although against these savings must be set the longer consultation times than in orthodox medicine. Evidence for economic benefit would be essential in any attempt to persuade the governments or insurance companies to reimburse the costs of homoeopathy. There are now constraints on spending in health services throughout the world. For example in Britain a recent leading article stated: 'The challenge (for health-care purchasers) is to substitute complementary medicine for conventional treatments rather than simply to add to the range of treatments and costs' (Smith, 1995). But every challenge can be seen as an opportunity. In the first place this is an opportunity for homoeopathy, to show that it can produce the same or even better care than current orthodox managements, and at a lower cost. Second, there is an opportunity in the fact that homoeopathy, in the UK at least, is often used to manage the sort of chronic patients whose needs are not currently being met by the health service, but who may cost considerable sums to society in terms of sickness benefit, lost production and so on. The potential opportunity for homoeopathy is to demonstrate that additional spending on health services will produce even greater financial benefits by reducing the other costs to society.

Economic evaluations can now be performed to rigorous standards thanks to two relatively recent advances. First, the quality of data recording has improved dramatically throughout health services, both because of computerization and in response to increasing awareness of the need to manage resources. Second, the methodology for economic evaluation has now become reasonably well established. The methods used were clearly set out in four strategic papers by Robinson (1993a–d). Drummond (1994), and Drummond and Jefferson (1996) have also been prominent in clarifying exactly what is required of an economic analysis, and recently set out full details of the criteria. This chapter will discuss some of the ways in which economic analysis can usefully be applied to homoeopathy.

Table 16.1

Analysis method	*Question posed*	*Example of outcome*
Cost-minimization	The outcome is fixed: which is the cheapest way of achieving it?	Hernia repair
Cost-effectiveness	Does a more expensive treatment have a greater effect on symptoms and signs?	Blood pressure reduction
Cost-utility	Which treatment is more acceptable to the patient, has greater effect on their quality of life?	SF-36
Cost-benefit	What is the balance between the treatment costs and their benefits (in ££)?	££ (e.g. drug costs)

Methodology

As with most medical specialties, economic evaluation has developed its own terminology which may appear to be a hindrance initially. It is essential to use the terms correctly so that a correct definition of the precise objective of the research can lead to an appropriate study design. The four basic methods will be described here and are set out in Table 16.1.

- *Cost-minimization* (or cost-comparison) might be used to compare a process such as provision of identical clinics in different situations; but there are few circumstances when the outcome of a homoeopathic treatment is precisely the same as that of an orthodox treatment and cost-minimization is probably not directly relevant to this discussion.
- It is *cost-effectiveness* analysis which would be used to compare the effect of homoeopathy with the effect of other treatments. For example homoeopathy could be compared with medication for symptomatic relief in hay-fever: 'Which treatment gives the greatest symptom relief per monetary unit?'
- *Cost-utility* analysis can be regarded as a refinement of cost-effectiveness. It was developed to guide the allocation of resources between differing diseases such as, say, cancer of the cervix and hypertension. Treatments are assessed in terms of their effect on a common measure, the QALY (quality adjusted life year) which is the result of multiplying the expected survival in years by the quality of life (on a scale of 0 to 1). This measure has to be broad with large measurement units in order to cover the whole range of disease, and it is not ideally suited to the conditions typically treated by homoeopathy. However, the idea behind the method is important for homoeopathy and is almost certainly more appropriate than cost-effectiveness analysis which only measures a single symptom and may ignore what is most useful for the patient (i.e. the 'utility' of the treatment). Homoeopathy may produce all sorts of other benefits, for example the improvement in apparently unrelated symptoms or the absence of adverse effects; these more subtle outcomes would be omitted in cost-effectiveness analysis but could be included in a cost-utility analysis.

The best ways of measuring the 'utility' of complementary medicine have not yet been agreed and the matter is discussed further in this chapter.

- The most comprehensive method of economic evaluation is *cost-benefit* analysis which produces a balance-sheet with the costs of treatment on one side, and the benefits in monetary terms on the other side. The viewpoint of the investigator will decide which benefits will be measured in the study: a purchaser of health care will consider it cost-beneficial if homoeopathic prescribing reduces drug costs, but the individual patient will want to know that the value of his/her symptom control is accounted for in the calculation! The approach that is most universally applicable is to consider society's overall viewpoint and include all possible costs and benefits. An example can be taken from the arguments in favour of manipulation. The annual cost to the UK health service of treating back pain is considerable (estimated to be half a billion pounds in 1993) and yet this is overshadowed by the costs to social security (£1.4 billion for benefit payments) and to industry (£3.8 billion in lost production) (Clinical Services Advisory Group, CSAG 1994). The Advisory Group calculated that an additional health intervention that produces a 1% reduction in the wider social costs of back pain would save £52m, and would therefore have a net cost benefit to society if it could be implemented for less than this amount.

Trial design

Although a number of economic analyses in orthodox medicine have been performed using published results of clinical trials, this approach is not ideal for homoeopathy since many of the costs will not be accessible and retrospective estimates will have to be made. The results of this kind of study may be of use in identifying areas for further research but will usually fail to provide definitive answers. There are strong arguments in favour of integrating economic analysis in controlled clinical trials: the costs that need to be measured can be established in advance with inclusion/exclusion criteria just like the clinical criteria, and they can be collected with objectivity and rigour in both the intervention and the control groups in parallel (Drummond, 1994). They remain secondary outcome measures, however, and do not detract from the integrity of the trial.

Since the medical and scientific communities have yet to be convinced that homoeopathy is effective for any particular indication, it is recommended that economic analysis trials of homoeopathy be double-blind and placebo-controlled. No other methodology can distinguish between the specific effects of homoeopathy and the non-specific effects of the overall 'package of care'. For example, a trial which compares homoeopathic management of myalgia with standard rheumatological care cannot draw conclusions about the cost-effectiveness of homoeopathy, only the cost-effectiveness of the whole combination of nutritional and lifestyle advice, therapeutic relationship and other non-specific effects in addition to any specific effects of the remedy. Results from such studies are not inherently generalizable. Rigorous double-blind studies of homoeopathy are eminently feasible since placebos can readily be produced that appear identical to the verum remedies.

Table 16.2 Questions that should be considered in the design of economic evaluation studies

What is the specific research question?
Is the question important?
Is the chosen method of evaluation appropriate?
Whose viewpoint(s) should be considered in the analysis?
Are the trial design and outcome measures appropriate?
Are all the expected costs accessible to measurement (or can good estimates be made of those which cannot be measured)?
Does the study have a good chance of answering the question?
Is the time-frame adequate to collect all the relevant data?
Has an attempt been made to identify all events which could seriously distort the results?

Once a particular remedy has been shown to be effective, one can proceed to studies which compare homoeopathy with orthodox management. The recommended procedure is to make comparisons with the cheapest, the most expensive and the most frequently used existing treatments.

A further essential feature of rigorous analyses is random allocation of the subjects to the intervention groups. It has been demonstrated that omitting randomization leads to an over-estimation of the effect of therapy by more than 40% on average (Schulz *et al.*, 1995). Randomization does not guarantee that prognostic factors are equally prevalent in the groups (unless stratified for such factors) but it does ensure that there is no systematic difference between the groups which would introduce bias. Randomization is undoubtedly the best way to make sure that the groups are in fact comparable in terms of known and unknown characteristics.

Patients may be less willing to be recruited to a study in which they may receive placebo, and clinicians may be uncomfortable knowing that they are prescribing placebos. The ethical justification for placebo trials of homoeopathy, however, is strong; namely that this is the only way to establish the efficacy of the treatment and is therefore in the best interests of patients in general. The 'optional cross-over' design (Ernst and Resch, 1995) was especially worked out to suit the needs of homoeopathy and makes placebo studies more acceptable; it will be discussed below.

Table 16.2 lists some questions which should be considered early in the planning stage of an economic analysis.

Examples of economic analysis of homoeopathy

In the UK, Swayne (1992) analysed computerized prescription records and showed that 22 homoeopathic primary care physicians working within the state health service issued 12% fewer prescriptions than the average for physicians in their area. The net mean ingredient cost was 30p less than the average. The author calculated that, if these savings were applied to prescription costs of the whole of the UK, the potential savings would be in the region of £69m per annum (at 1992 rates).

In 1984, Feldhaus introduced *Arnica montana 12X* routinely into his dental practice, prescribing it for 3 days before and 7 days after dental

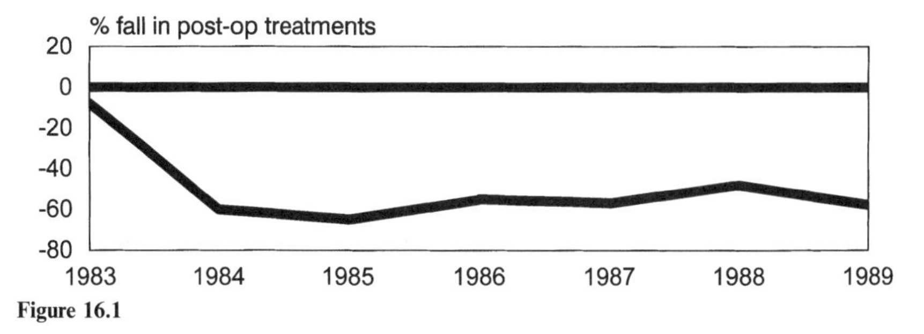

Figure 16.1

surgery (Feldhaus, 1993). Using the records of claims for health insurance payments, he reviewed the incidence of postoperative complications for one year before and 7 years after the introduction. As shown in Figure 16.1, the complication rate fell to 40% below the average for other dentists in the region. This resulted in estimated annual savings of DM1209 in insurance company payouts. The number of sickness certificates issued fell by approximately the same percentage. There are several possible explanations for this finding besides the suggested effect of *Arnica,* such as alterations in dental technique and skills of auxiliary personnel. However, this is an important claim and a suitable topic for a more rigorous investigation.

Wiesenauer *et al.* (1992) also performed an analysis by examining the insurance records of treatment costs, this time of 87 doctors who use the title 'naturopath' or 'homoeopath'. The authors compared the costs of 97 doctors who do not use these titles. Drug costs were 15% lower in the naturopath/homoeopath group, which was statistically significant. Overall treatment costs were measured on a points system and were 8.2% lower in the naturopath/homoeopath group, which was not significant but represents a cost saving of DM2.6 per patient.

All these trials suffer from considerable methodological limitations. First, they are all retrospective and non-randomized, therefore the two groups which were being compared are unlikely to have been comparable in all important characteristics. For example, people who visited the homoeopaths may have been less ill, and there is evidence that they would be more likely to have positive attitudes towards a healthy lifestyle (Furnham and Bhagrath, 1993). Second, outcomes are not measured so the effectiveness of treatments, clearly a major consideration to the patients, is ignored. Therefore these studies can only provide a cost-benefit analysis purely from the point of view of the health purchaser.

Outcome measures

The primary outcome measure must be appropriate for the particular purpose of the economic analysis. Simple measures of change ('slightly better', 'much better' etc.) may reflect the patients' wish to please the doctor as much as any real alterations in the condition and are best avoided except as supplementary questions.

Cost-effectiveness requires a single robust but 'natural' measure of effectiveness such as days off work or analgesic consumption. *Cost-utility* studies attempt to measure the impact of treatment in a more holistic way. Quality of life in orthodox cost-utility research is measured on the Rosser Index and more recently the EuroQol (Williams, 1995) measure, both of which have gradations of scale that are probably too large to be sensitive enough for the changes likely to be seen after homoeopathy. The Nottingham Health Profile is a validated measure which measures health in a range of dimensions (Jenkinson, 1994) and was used to examine cost-benefit of acupuncture in stroke patients, albeit in a very limited analysis (Johansson *et al.*, 1993). However Brazier *et al.* (1992) showed that the newly-developed Short Form with 36 questions (SF-36) can identify smaller degrees of impaired health than the Nottingham Health Profile, and its validity and change over time have been established. However its time frame of four weeks is rather long for some conditions, and up to 25% of patients have difficulty completing it. Another drawback for its use in economic analysis is that it was not designed to generate a single index figure for quality of life, since the eight different areas of enquiry are not measured on an ordinal scale, nor is the relation between them known. Thus there is no way of comparing the values of large changes in (say) physical functioning and in mental health.

These newly developed measures attempt to move away from just measuring symptoms and try to reflect what the patient him/herself feels is important for his/her health. Homoeopaths would have sympathy with this intention. One of the most refined techniques in this area is the Schedule for the Evaluation of Individual Quality of Life (SEIQoL), in which patients choose the five 'dimensions' which are most important for them and then assess the impact the illness has had on these areas (McGee *et al.,* 1991). This instrument is still under development and has the serious disadvantage of relying on interviews which are expensive.

There is also considerable interest in the MYMOP measure (Measure Your own Medical Outcome Profile) in which subjects are asked first to nominate their worst one or two symptoms and score them on a Likert-type scale, and second to score how much impact these symptoms are having on a (nominated) activity of daily living. Paterson showed that MYMOP is valid in comparison with the SF-36 and appears to be more sensitive to the sorts of changes one is likely to see in complementary medicine (Paterson, 1996). However, it has been argued that it is superficial, and although it may appear more sensitive than the SF-36 it is not measuring underlying changes in health which are important for the patient (Jenkinson, 1996). It was also pointed out that there is no logical justification for combining the scores of the different questions into a single 'profile'.

It is worth considering whether any measure which assesses *function* might include a kind of proxy assessment of the utility of treatment, given the overriding importance of function in life: for example the Oswestry scale for back pain (Fairbank *et al.*, 1980) involves answering practical questions such as the length of time the patient can sit in any chair before having to get up. None of these outcome measures have yet been shown to be validated for economic evaluation, but they appear to be the best available measures and it is important to start to gain experience with them if only to stimulate debate and develop better measures.

An entirely different approach to the problem of measuring 'soft' endpoints and 'patient preference' is through a novel methodology called 'optional cross-ever' design (Ernst and Resch, 1995). Subjects are initially allocated at random to intervention and control groups in the usual way, but at a later consultation any subject who feels he/she is not improving is given the chance to cross over into the opposite treatment group. After another treatment period he/she is given a second opportunity to cross back again to the first group. This may happen as many times as is predetermined until the cut-point, when the primary endpoint is measured, i.e. the proportion of subjects ending up in each group. This design is not disease-specific and offers a single common endpoint which can be used to assess patients' responses in a variety of conditions in a single situation. It is clearly not appropriate for short-term or self-limiting conditions. Economic analysis of such a trial would begin measuring benefits only after the cut-point.

Thus it can be seen that there is no clear outcome measure yet developed which measures what the patient regards as important, produces a single figure to compare different conditions, and is appropriate for conditions seen in homoeopathy.

Cost-benefit assesses the costs and effects of treatment in terms of hard cash: 'How much did the homoeopathic treatment cost and how much was it worth?' Clearly it is difficult to assess the value of a reduction in symptoms in monetary terms, although special techniques are available such as 'willingness to pay' (Thompson, 1986). USA residents were interviewed and it was concluded that they would be prepared to pay about 20% of their domestic income for a cure for arthritis. Conversion of quality of life data into financial value is still in the early stages of research and is unlikely to be applied to the field of homoeopathy for some time. The cost-saving of early return to work is also problematic, although national norms have been established. In practice it is likely to be drug, consultation and referral costs which are more readily accessible, although an analysis that uses these outcomes alone will produce a result that is rather limited in perspective, i.e. the costs of the health service purchaser.

Measuring costs

Table 16.3 lists the categories in which costs may need to be collected in an economic analysis. These costs should be defined before the study commences, with inclusion/exclusion criteria just like the clinical criteria for defining the population to be treated. In practice some costs are notoriously difficult to measure accurately, yet they may be very relevant to the assessment (e.g. patients' costs for repeated attendance for homoeopathy). Where national standards are not available estimates may be made but this should be stated. It is preferable to make both high and low estimates and to repeat the calculations with both thus giving an estimate of the confidence of the result. This process is one simple form of 'sensitivity analysis' (Coyle and Davies, 1993).

Table 16.3 Categories of treatment costs which should be considered

Direct medical costs/ intervention costs	*Service costs*	*Direct non-medical costs*	*Indirect morbidity costs*
Practioner fees and expenses	Rental of clinic rooms (or capital costs), heat and light	Transport costs, including relatives	Loss of time from work or caring for family
Diagnostic costs: X-rays, etc.	Ancillary staff, including nurse, etc.		Cost of caring e.g. relatives' loss of time from work
Therapy costs: needles, etc.	Office costs including computers, stationery		Stress, pain, etc.
Costs borne by the patient (analgesics, dressings, etc.)		Costs borne by society	

'Induced' costs of subsequent treatments, including management of adverse reactions, should be considered in the analysis

Economic evaluation methodology has developed its own terminology to express concepts which are peculiar to itself. Two examples are 'opportunity' and 'marginal' costs. Opportunity costs should ideally be used for staff and equipment, i.e. of the cost of their next most efficient use if they were not employed in the study. However, actual market costs are adequate in most cases. It is usually appropriate to measure the marginal costs and benefits which represent expansion or contraction at the margins of a service that is already provided. Marginal costs are likely to be different from average costs. For example, expensive investigations are likely to be performed soon after admission for stroke and will be included in calculating the average costs of a patient's admission; but alterations to the duration of stay will only alter therapist and 'hotel' costs, in which case the marginal costs will be lower than average costs.

Sample size

The required sample size for economic evaluation studies can be calculated from knowledge about the endpoints in the usual way, even if the outcome is a unit of currency rather than a measurement of symptoms: larger samples will be needed if there is much scatter in the measurements of the endpoint (i.e. large standard deviation), and smaller samples will be sufficient if there is expected to be a considerable difference in outcome between the groups. For example, the disease episode in acute self-limiting conditions is likely to be short, symptoms may be very variable between individuals, and interventions may have only a small impact: in this case large numbers of patients are likely to be required. Therefore figures for the chosen outcome (whether quality of life, pain scores, drug costs, etc.) should be obtained from existing records, from a small pilot study or from published research in the area. The required sample size is then calculated using a formula or computer program. Studies which do not have adequate numbers of subjects risk producing false negative or false positive results.

Analysing the data

The final economic analysis is simply a question of calculation. However, if the costs or the benefits are likely to last more than 12 months it is usual to consider 'discounting' which reflects the fact that next year's benefit isn't worth quite as much as this year's because it has been delayed by a year. Robinson (1993b) gives the necessary references, and the question is further discussed by Drummond (1994).

It is a good general principle that research reports should include sufficient data to allow readers to repeat the inferential statistics and test the data in different ways. Drummond (1994) emphasizes the particular need for reporting the raw data in economic analyses since the information itself may then be reinterpreted by other specialists, for instance to suggest hypotheses from a different perspective. It is acknowledged that early reports will be in some sense primitive since this a groundbreaking area of research. In particular the information collected may be limited but it is essential that this work is published in order to allow progress to be made.

Finally, the report should include some assessment of how generalizable the results are, bearing in mind differences in local costs, practice procedures, patient age group and so on. Again it should be noted that there are limits to generalizing from a study that is not randomized or placebo-controlled because the practitioner may be providing an important input into the patient's improvement and this will inevitably be different with another practitioner.

Conclusion

There are no rigorous studies of the economic effects of homoeopathy yet very good reasons exist to conduct such research. The methodology is now defined, and clear analysis of the aims of the research will lead to appropriate trial design and the measurement of the correct endpoints. Early attempts at economic evaluation may provide incomplete data or have other problems which have not been anticipated but this should not deter investigators since such studies are crucial for developing better methods to research this critically important area.

References

Brazier, J.E., Harper, R., Jones, N.M.B. *et al.* (1992) Validating the SF-36 health survey questionnaire: new outcome measure for primary care. *Brit. Med. J.*, **305**, 160–64.

Coyle, D. and Davies, L. (1993) How to assess cost-effectiveness: elements of a sound economic evaluation. In *Purchasing and providing cost-effective health care* (M.F. Drummond and A. Maynard, eds) pp. 66–79, Churchill Livingstone.

CSAG 1994 Committee Report: Back Pain. HMSO London.

Drummond, M. (1994) Economic analysis alongside controlled trials. R&D Directorate, Quarry House, Quarry Hill, Leeds, UK.

Drummond, M. and Jefferson, T.O. (1996) Guidelines for authors and peer reviewers of economic submissions to the BMJ. *Brit. Med. J.*, **313**, 275–83.

Ernst, E. and Resch, K.L. (1995) The 'optional cross-over design' for randomized controlled trials. *Fundam. Clin. Pharmacol.*, **9**, 508–11.

Fairbank, J.C.T., Couper, J., Davies, J.B. and O'Brien, J.P. (1980) The Oswestry low back pain disability questionnaire. *Physiotherapy*, **66**(8), 271–3.

Feldhaus, H.-W. (1993) Cost-effectiveness of homoeopathic treatment in a dental practice. *British Homoeopathic Journal*, **82**, 22–8.

Furnham, A. and Bhagrath, R. (1993) A comparison of health beliefs and behaviours of clients of orthodox and complementary medicine. *Brit. J. Clin. Psychol.*, **32**, 237–46.

Jenkinson, C. (1994) Weighting for ill-health: the Nottingham Health Profile. In *Measuring Health and Medical Outcomes* (C. Jenkinson, ed.) pp. 77–88, UCL Press.

Jenkinson, C. (1996) MYMOP, a patient generated measure of outcomes [letter]. *Brit. Med. J.*, **313**, 626.

Johansson, K., Lindgren, I., Widner, H. *et al.* (1993) Can sensory stimulation improve the functional outcome in stroke patients? *Neurology*, **43**, 2189–92.

McGee, H.M., O'Boyle, C.A., Hickey, A. *et al.* (1991) Assessing the quality of life of the individual: the SEIQoL with a healthy and a gastroenterology unit population. *Psychol. Med.*, **21**, 749–59.

Paterson, C. (1996) Measuring outcomes in primary care: a patient-generated measure, MYMOP, compared with the SF-36 health survey. *Brit. Med. J.*, **312**, 1016–20.

Robinson, R. (1993a) Economic evaluation and health care: what does it mean? *Brit. Med. J.*, **307**, 670–73.

Robinson, R. (1993b) Costs and cost-minimization analysis. *Brit. Med. J.*, **307**, 726–8.

Robinson, R. (1993c) Cost-effectiveness analysis. *Brit. Med. J.*, **307**, 793–5.

Robinson, R. (1993d) Cost-utility analysis. *Brit. Med. J.*, **307**, 859–62.

Robinson, R. (1993e) Cost-benefit analysis. *Brit. Med. J.*, **307**, 924–6.

Schulz, K.F., Chalmers, I., Hayes, R.J. and Altman, D.G. (1995) Empirical evidence of bias. *JAMA*, **273**(5), 408–12.

Smith, I. (1995) Commissioning complementary medicine. *Brit. Med. J.*, **310**, 1151–2.

Swayne, J. (1992) The cost and effectiveness of homoeopathy. *British Homoeopathic Journal*, **81**, 148–50.

Thompson, M.S. (1986) Willingness to pay and accept risks to cure chronic diseases. *Am. J. Public Health*, **76**(4), 392–6.

Wiesenauer, M., Groh, P. and Häussler, S. (1992) Naturheilkunde asl Beitrag zur Kostendämpfung. *Forsch. Komplementärmed.*, **17**, 311–14.

Williams, A. (1995) The role of the EuroQol instrument in QALY calculations. Discussion Paper 130, Centre for Health Economics, University of York, UK. 1996.

Chapter 17

Socioeconomic aspects of homoeopathy as seen by decision-takers and service providers in the public health system

Benno Brinkhaus, Gernot Schindler, Martin Lindner, Alexandra Jansen and Eckhart G. Hahn

Introduction

Over the last two decades, the demand for complementary medical treatment and diagnostic procedures has increased worldwide. Thus, in 1990, in the USA the number of consultations in the field of complementary medicine (425 million) exceeded those in the entire field of orthodox primary care medicine (388 million consultations) (Eisenberg *et al.*, 1993). In Europe, the use of complementary medicine by the population varies between 10% (Denmark) and 49% (France) (Aldridge, 1989; Knipschild, Kleijnen and ter Riet, 1990). Studies on the use of complementary medicine done in the USA, Canada, New Zealand and Australia show that the constantly increasing numbers of such treatments is a worldwide phenomenon (Clinical Oncology Group, 1987; Eisenberg *et al.*, 1993; Marshall *et al.*, 1990; Northcott and Bachynsky, 1993; Thomas, Westlake and Williams, 1991; Yates *et al.*, 1993). In parallel with the increasing use of complementary medical diagnostic and therapeutic methods in the USA and Europe, the unconventional treatment modality of homoeopathy is also being employed ever more frequently (Fisher, 1994). Thus, in Europe, between 15% and 56% of the population makes additional or alternative use of homoeopathy to supplement conventional treatment of a range of illnesses (Fisher, 1994). In France, the use of homoeopathic diagnostic and therapeutic methods increased from 16% in 1982, to 36% in 1992 (L'Homéopathie en 1993, cited by Fisher, 1994). In Belgium, 85% of the general practitioners also offer homoeopathy as a complementary therapeutic modality (Aldridge, 1989; Knipschild, Kleijnen and ter Riet, 1990).

In parallel with the increasing use of complementary medical diagnostic and therapeutic procedures, in the USA and the EU countries, the costs of such treatments are also rising (Eisenberg *et al.*, 1993; Fisher, 1994). For the most part, these costs have to be met by the patients themselves. In 1990, in the USA three-quarters of the costs of complementary medicine treatments (US $10.3 billion) were defrayed by the patients themselves (Eisenberg *et al.*, 1993). Also in the EU countries, the costs of complementary medicine have for the most part to be paid, albeit to varying extents, by the patients themselves (Fisher, 1994). This also applies to homoeopathy, where, as a rule, neither the often time-consuming initial medical consultation, nor the homoeopathic remedies, are paid for by the state health insurance carriers.

In recent years, this situation has increasingly prompted patients to demand of political decision-takers and the cost carriers (health insurance carriers, care-providing institutions) that the costs of complementary medical treatments (including homoeopathy) should be reimbursed. An epidemiological survey revealed that approximately 60% of the German population would employ complementary medicine, provided that the state or health insurance carriers paid for the treatment (Repräsentativumfrage im Auftrage der Innungskrankenkassenbundes 1993, cited by Schüppel, 1994).

In contrast, the representatives of health insurance carriers and politicians are adopting a more skeptical stance towards the financing of complementary medical methods. Against the background of increasing health care costs, those with responsibility within the public health sector, draw attention to the lack of financial resources. Thus, for example, in the EU countries, expenditure for direct health-related services expressed as a percentage of the gross national product increased between 1980 and 1990 from 7.11% to 7.85% and in the USA from 8.25% to 11.02% (Schneider *et al.*, 1993). In addition, those with responsibility for the public health system are increasingly pointing to the general lack of proof of the effectiveness of complementary medical methods.

As a complementary medical mode of treatment, homoeopathy has, over the last two decades, increasingly been the subject of clinical scientific studies aimed at investigating its effects (Kleijnen, Knipschild and ter Riet, 1991; Linde *et al.*, 1995). These studies have shown a tendency for homoeopathy to produce positive effects in selected indications (Kleijnen, Knipschild and ter Riet, 1991). However, most of the clinical scientific studies so far carried out have been of poor quality in terms of their methodology (Ernst, 1995; Fisher, 1994; Kleijnen, Knipschild and ter Riet, 1991).

Against this background, politicians and economists are demanding more scientific research into these unconventional methods, including homoeopathy, and a number of specific research programmes are currently being funded. Thus, for example, in December 1993, the project 'Homoeopathic Medicine in Europe' was initiated, with the aim of promoting a greater international research effort into the therapeutic methods of homoeopathy (Fisher, 1994). In Germany, the Ministry for Research and Education (BMBF) initiated the project 'Unkonventionelle Medizinische Richtungen' (Unconventional Therapeutic Methods). The aim of this project is to intensify the scientific research effort into complementary medical methods including homoeopathy (Matthiessen, 1992).

The contradiction between the increasing use of and expenditure on complementary medicine on the one hand, and the restrictive attitudes of cost carriers in the public health sector on the other, is striking, and, in view of the increasing sociopolitical and economic importance of the problems involved, requires detailed analysis.

In an attempt to determine the sociopolitical and socioeconomic status quo of the complementary medical method of homoeopathy, we carried out an epidemiological study in five EU countries, to interview decision-takers and service providers in the public health sector who on the basis of their medical, political or scientific activities are experts in the socioeconomic aspects of public health care. At the same time, as a result of their professional activities, this group of individuals is at the cutting edge of development and research in the area of complementary medicine, in that they can determine the future direction, and even the fate, of alternative medicine.

Methods

The present epidemiological study was conducted between March and June, 1996, by the Research Group for Traditional and Complementary Medicine at the Department of Medicine I at the Friedrich-Alexander University in Erlangen.

The target groups of the epidemiological study were directors of university medical departments, politicians, editors of medical journals, representatives of the pharmaceutical industry and representatives of health insurance carriers, general practitioners and homoeopaths. From a single pool of all the potential target addresses, the representatives of the target groups who were finally approached, were selected using a defined random code taking acount of the target parameters occupational group and country. Finally, a total of 1577 individuals in the target groups in the five EU countries, Austria, Belgium, France, Germany and Great Britain were interviewed using a postal questionnaire. All those approached were informed as to the objective, method and purpose of the study, which was conducted in such a way as to ensure the anonymity of all responders.

Before designing the questionnaire, an intensive search of the current literature (Medline, Embase, DHU-database) was carried out to obtain information of relevance for deciding the content and formal definition of the items in the questionnaire. The final questions were then vetted by an international team of experts. For the most part, the questionnaire contained closed questions, but also a number of opportunities for the interviewee's own remarks. The closed questions were formally of the question and answer type providing simple alternatives (yes/no) or multiple choices, unstructured multiple choices, multiple answers and seven-step scales. Each questionnaire received a separate registration number, and the items in the questionnaire were translated into English, French and Dutch by native speakers.

The following defined points were used to determine, among other things, the socioeconomic position of homoeopathy in the EU countries:

- age, sex, occupation/profession, residence (country) and field of activity of the interviewee;
- value of homoeopathy within the public health sector;
- reimbursement of the costs of homoeopathic treatments by the health insurance carriers;
- willingness to pay privately for homoeopathic treatment;
- the influence of a greater use of homoeopathy on cost developments in the public health sector;
- results of homoeopathic treatments used for a range of indications.

In a pilot survey, the initial version of the questionnaire, in German, was critically investigated for ease of understanding of the questions, the relevance of the formal design, and the time taken to complete the questionnaire. Four weeks after distribution of the first questionnaire, a postal reminder was sent to the interviewees with the aim of increasing the response rate. Twelve weeks after dispatching the first questionnaire and eight weeks after posting the reminder, the data bank was closed. The returned questionnaires were documented and the data submitted for statistical evaluation.

The documentation was carried out by the Research Group for Complementary Medicine (Department of Medicine I) at the University of Erlangen-Nuremberg. The software employed for this purpose was the Statistical Package for Social Science (SPSS) Version 6.1.3. The Department for Biometry and Medical Documentation at the University of Ulm performed the statistical analysis of the data using the software Statistical Analysis System (SAS) Version 6.08. The statistical evaluation was conducted with the aid of frequency and contingency tables.

For a descriptive analysis we defined three groups – supporters of homoeopathy, opponents of homoeopathy, and those indifferent to homoeopathy – on the basis of a variable classification of items (efficacy of homoeopathy, willingness to pay for homoeopathic treatment privately, personal use of homoeopathy, satisfaction/dissatisfaction with personal homoeopathic treatment in general, and satisfaction/dissatisfaction with the outcome of personal treatment in particular).

Results

The response rate was 33.8% (n = 533). The responders were 25.1% female, 74.1% male; the average age of the responders was 50.2 (± 10,7) years. From the responders 41.1% had frequent, 35.7% occasional and 21.8% no contact with homoeopathy (Table 17.1).

Among the occupational groups, the most frequent responses came from directors of university medical departments (51%), homoeopaths (43%) and politicians (36%). In contrast, the response rate was below average among representatives of the pharmaceutical industry (27%), general practitioners (25%), representatives of health insurance carriers (25%) and editors of medical journals (23%). With respect to the countries involved, the response rate was highest in Austria (44%) and Germany (42%), followed by Great Britain and Belgium (31% each) and finally France (23%). Of the responders, in accordance with the above-mentioned criteria, 35% were classified as supporters, 29% as opponents of homoeopathy, while 36% remained indifferent to homoeopathy. Among the homoeopaths, supporters of homoeopathy predominated (76%); among the directors of university medical departments in contrast, the majority were opponents (70%). Among all the other occupational groups, those indifferent to homoeopathy were in the majority.

Value of homoeopathy in the health system

The assessment of the usefulness of homoeopathy by all responders was balanced in terms of the answers 'very great' (23%), 'great' (18%), 'moderate' (19%) to 'slight' (21%). A small number (9%) of the responders saw 'no value' in homoeopathy, considered it to be 'harmful' (3%) or expressed no opinion on this question 'don't know' (7%) (Figure 17.1).

Table 17.1 Characteristics of respondents

		%	n
Decision makers	Addressees	100.0	1577
	Respondents	33.8	533
Gender	Male	74.1	395
	Female	25.1	134
Age in years (m ± s)		50.2 ± 10.7	
Residence	Austria	14.6	78
	Belgium	9.6	51
	France	16.5	88
	Germany	37.7	201
	United Kingdom	21.6	115
Professions	General practitioners	17.1	91
	Homoeopaths	29.4	157
	University-directors	22.7	121
	Pharmaceutical industries	17.1	91
	Politicians	4.9	26
	Editors	3.5	19
	Health insurance carriers	5.3	28
Occupational contact with homoeopathy	Exclusively	13.1	70
	Very often	16.7	89
	Often	11.4	61
	Occasionally	35.7	190
	Never	21.8	116
	Missings	1.3	7

Large differences are to be seen between the views of responding homoeopaths and directors of university medical departments in this question: the homoeopaths very frequently (86%) assessed the value of homoeopathy to be 'very great' or 'great', while the directors of university medical departments most frequently considered it to be of only 'slight' (48%) or 'moderate' (13%) value. This occupational group also most commonly assessed homoeopathy to be of 'no value' (24%) or 'harmful' (9%). Over and beyond this, in terms of the percentage response rates to this question, replies by the homoeopaths showed virtually identical distributions to those of the supporters of homoeopathy, and this also applied to the directors of university medical departments in comparison with the opponents of homoeopathy.

In the same context the other five occupational groups approached showed only small differences. General practitioners least often considered homoeopathy to be of value (27% considering it to be of 'very great' or 'great' value, 52% of 'moderate' or 'slight' value, while politicians most commonly believed it to be of value (39% and 50%, respectively). In common with the directors of university medical departments, the editors of medical journals most frequently opted for the answers 'no value' and 'harmful' (16% and 5%, respectively).

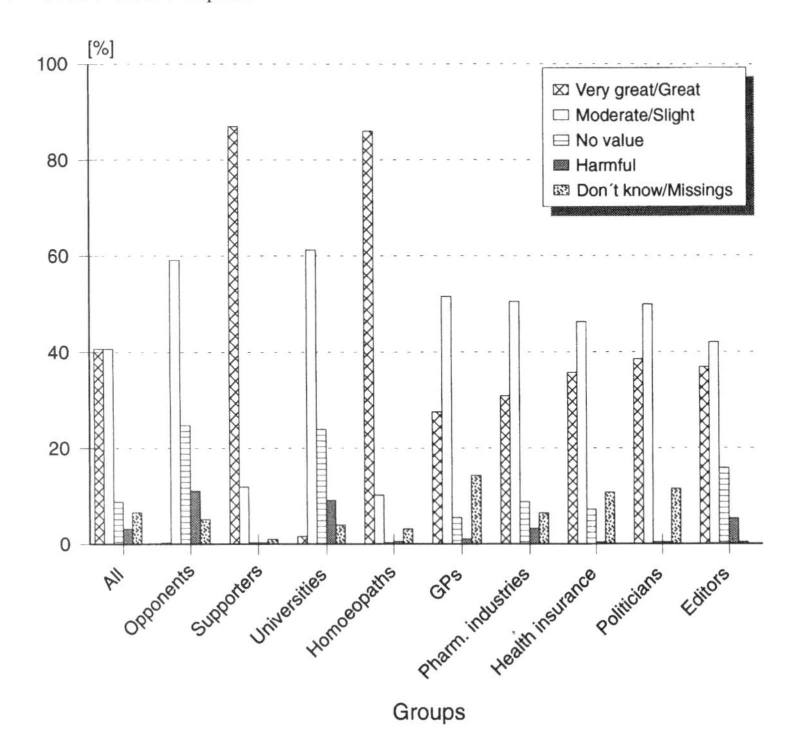

Figure 17.1 Value of homoeopathy in the health system.

Payment of costs of homoeopathic treatment by the health insurance carriers

A majority of all responders (40%) favoured payment of homoeopathic treatment by the health insurance carriers; almost one-third (30%) were in favour of payment in part, while 23% rejected such payment outright. Of those questioned, 7% expressed no opinion (Figure 17.2).

The majority (62%) of the directors of university medical departments rejected full payment of such treatment, while approximately one-quarter (26%) favoured payment in part. In contrast, a small minority (5%) of this occupational group did favour full payment of homoeopathic treatment by the health insurance carriers. In comparison, the majority (76%) of the homoeopaths favoured full payment, and almost one-fifth (19%) for payment in part of homoeopathy by the health insurance carriers. None of the responding homoeopaths rejected the idea of reimbursement of the costs of homoeopathic treatment by the health insurance carriers. In this question, too, the percentage distributions of the answers among the opponents of homoeopathy were virtually identical with those of the directors of university medical departments, while this was also true of the supporters of homoeopathy and homoeopaths.

Among the occupational groups, representatives of the health insurance carriers and the politicians most commonly (50% and 42% respectively) favoured payment of homoeopathic treatment by the health insurance

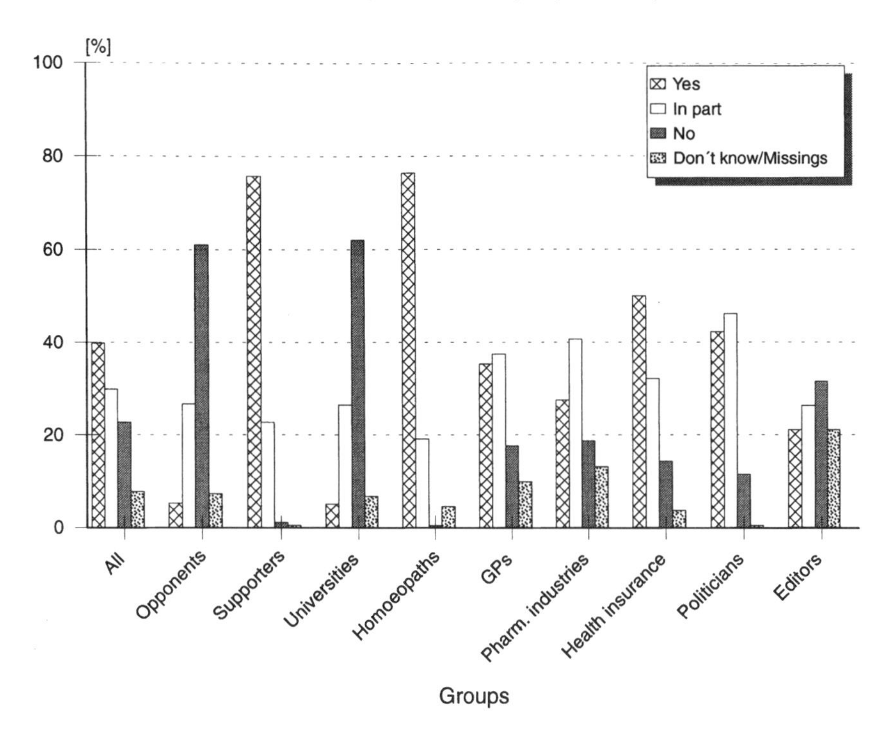

Figure 17.2 Payment of cost of homoeopathic treatment by the health insurance carriers.

carriers, and rejected such payment least often (14% and 12% respectively). In contrast, the occupational group that most often rejected such payment (32%), or by far the most frequently had no opinion (21%), were the editors.

Willingness to pay for homoeopathic treatment privately

The majority of all responders (54%) showed a willingness to pay for homoeopathic treatment out of their own pockets if the health insurance carriers would not do so. Approximately one-third (35%) of all those approached were not prepared to pay for homoeopathic treatment themselves, while some 10% had no opinion ('don't know') on this (Figure 17.3).

A minority (12%) of the directors of university medical departments and of the general practitioners (38%) expressed their willingness to pay for homoeopathic treatment privately. In contrast, more than one-half of the editors and representatives of the pharmaceutical industry (53% each) were prepared to pay for such treatment out of their own pockets. By far the greatest readiness to pay for homoeopathic therapy privately was shown by the homoeopaths (92%), followed by the politicians (69%) and the representatives of the health insurance carriers (64%).

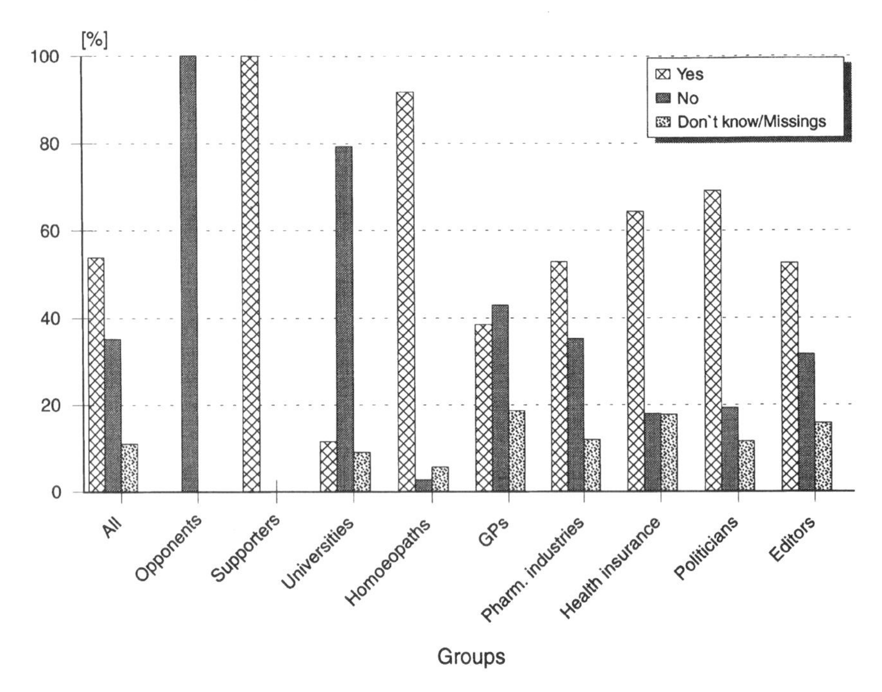

Figure 17.3 Willingness to pay for homoeopathic treatment privately.

Influence of a greater use of homoeopathy on costs in the public health sector

Of all those responding, the majority (55%) were of the opinion that increased use of homoeopathy could potentially result in a reduction in the costs of the health service (first three steps on the seven-step scale). Almost one-quarter of the responders (24%) took the opposite view (last three steps on the seven-step scale) (Figure 17.4).

Most of the directors of university medical departments (53%) were of the opinion that increased use of homoeopathy could not reduce health care costs. This opinion was shared by just under one-quarter (24%) of the general practitioners. The majority of the supporters of homoeopathy (96%), the homoeopaths (92%) and the politicians (73%) considered that a reduction in the costs of the public health system through the use of homoeopathy might be possible. Of the seven occupational groups approached, five (directors of university medical departments, general practitioners, representatives of the pharmaceutical industry, the health insurance carriers and editors) relatively frequently (> 20%) had no opinion on this point (answer: 'don't know').

Use of homoeopathy to treat various indications

In the view of the majority of responders, homoeopathy can be used most successfully to treat functional disorders (68%) and chronic illnesses (63%) (Figure 17.5). In contrast, appreciably fewer responders considered

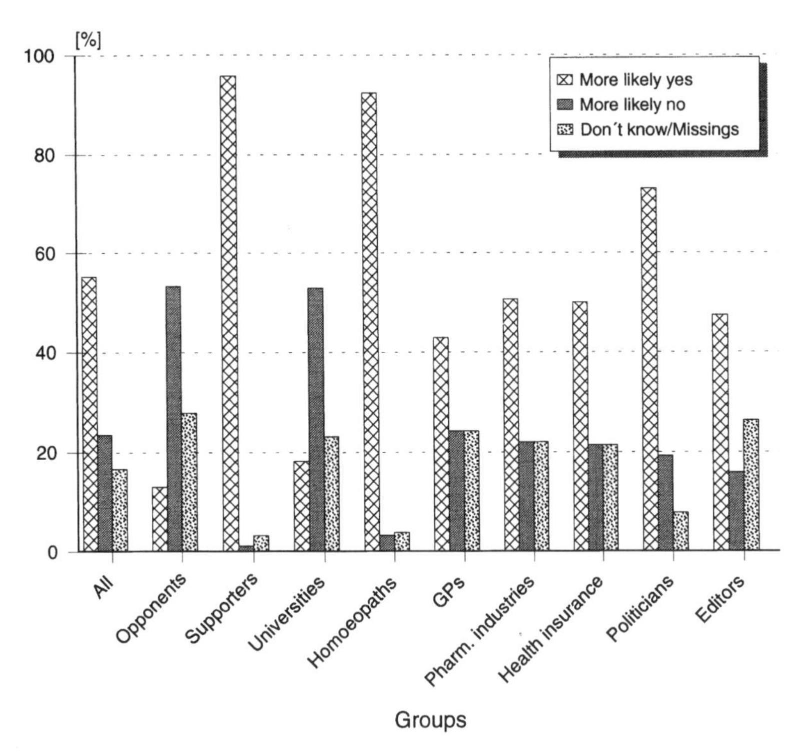

Figure 17.4 Influence of a greater use of homoeopathy on the development of costs in the public health sector.

homoeopathy capable of successfully treating psychiatric illnesses (43%) or acute conditions (38%) – only a small percentage of the respondents (7%) were of the opinion that none of the disorders/illnesses listed in the questionnaire would be amenable to homoeopathic treatment. A virtually identical percentage (8%) believed that additional disorders/illnesses (in particular psychosomatic and immunological disorders) could be successfully treated with homoeopathy. Just under one-half (48%) of the opponents of homoeopathy believed that functional complaints could be treated successfully by homoeopathic means. Only a rather small percentage of the opponents of homoeopathy considered that psychiatric and chronic illnesses could be successfully treated (20% and 19%, respectively), and only a tiny percentage (1%) thought acute diseases to be an indication for homoeopathy. One-fifth (20%) of all the opponents of homoeopathy were of the opinion that none of the illnesses listed could be treated successfully with homoeopathy.

The majority of its supporters considered that homoeopathy might be successfully used to treat all of the disorders/illnesses listed. In the case of chronic disorders (99%) and functional diseases (92%) in particular, treatment was considered likely to be successful. In addition, most supporters believed that both acute (82%) and psychiatric conditions (70%) would respond to homoeopathic treatment.

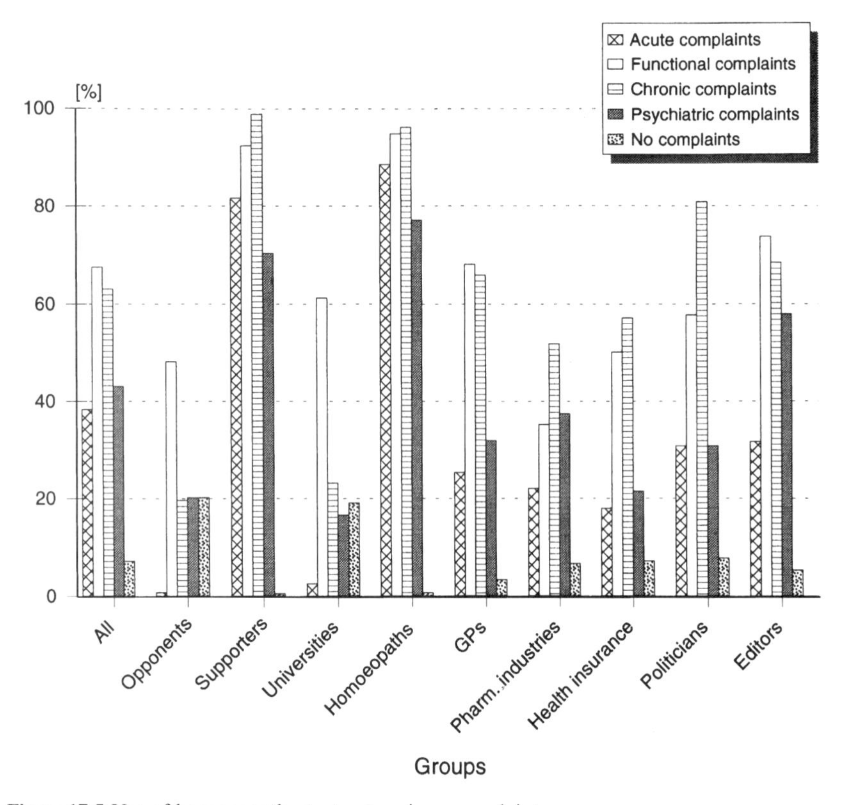

Figure 17.5 Use of homoeopathy to treat various complaints.

Most of the directors of university medical departments (61%) considered that functional illnesses might respond positively to homoeopathic treatment. Far fewer (23% and 17%) believed that chronic and psychiatric illnesses might respond to homoeopathic treatment. A percentage (19%) of the directors of university medical departments comparable with that of the opponents of homoeopathy took the view that none of the disorders/illnesses listed would respond positively to homoeopathic treatment.

The majority of the homoeopaths were of the opinion that chronic (96%), functional (95%), acute (89%) and psychiatric illnesses (77%) are all amenable to homoeopathic treatment.

Discussion

The results of the present epidemiological study show that decision-takers and opinion-formers in the public health sector differ considerably in their assessment of the therapeutic value of homoeopathy, and thus of the social benefits of this mode of treatment.

Thus, the majority of all respondents were of the opinion that functional (68%) and chronic (63%) diseases could be successfully treated with the complementary medical treatment homoeopathy. In contrast, psychiatric and acute diseases were considered to be less amenable to treatment with homoeopathy (43% and 38% of all respondents, respectively). With respect to the assessments by the occupational groups, clear differences were to be seen in terms of frequencies of response between supporters of homoeopathy/homoeopaths on the one hand, and opponents of homoeopathy/directors of university medical departments on the other. The former were convinced that homoeopathy is highly successful in the treatment of chronic (99%/96%) and functional (92%/95%) illnesses. In the view of this group, psychiatric (70%/89%) and acute (82%/77%) illnesses can also be successfully treated with homoeopathy. These high frequencies of response from the supporters of homoeopathy and homoeopaths with respect to indications for homoeopathy suggest a high level of satisfaction with homoeopathy as a therapeutic principle, or great confidence in the effectiveness of this treatment modality. In contrast, opponents of homoeopathy/directors of university medical departments believed that homoeopathy is a therapeutic principle with but little effect (functional diseases: 48%/61%; chronic diseases: 19%/23%; psychiatric conditions: 20%/17%).

At present, functional illnesses could not be successfully treated over the long-term with conventional therapies (Klein, 1988). The relatively high percentages of opponents of homoeopathy/directors of university medical departments who considered functional diseases – as opposed to other, organic disease groups – to be amenable to homoeopathic treatment reflect their view that homoeopathy has an unspecific/placebo effect rather than an organic pharmacological action. This confirms the commonly held assessment of representatives of conventional medicine, namely that homoeopathy produces no real measurable results, but must be considered merely to offer hope or to represent a 'last-ditch' attempt at treatment when all else has failed.

This is also confirmed by the data on the assessment of the value of homoeopathy. Thus, both supporters of homoeopathy and homoeopaths not only expressed a high level of satisfaction with homoeopathy in a variety of indications, but also felt it would be of considerable benefit within the health care system. In contrast, opponents of homoeopathy/directors of university medical departments were of the opinion that homoeopathy would be of only moderate (13%/13%) or slight (46%/48%) value within the health care sector.

With respect to the reimbursement of the costs of homoeopathic treatment by the health insurance carriers, 40% of the respondents favoured complete payment of such treatment by the health insurance carriers, 30% were in favour of payment in part, while just under one-quarter (23%) completely rejected any such payment. This reflects the estimation of the value of homoeopathy within the health care system, with 41% of the responders considering the value of homoeopathy to be very great or great, 40% believing it to be moderate or slight, and 9% attributing no value to it. Accordingly and consistently, only about one-half of all the responders (55%) thought that the use of homoeopathy could reduce costs in the public health sector.

Three-quarters of supporters/homoeopaths (76%/76%) favoured complete payment of homoeopathic treatment costs by the health insurance carriers. Furthermore, the majority of homoeopaths (92%) were prepared to pay for homoeopathic treatment out of their own pockets. These high percentages occasion no surprise, since the homoeopaths considered homoeopathy to be highly effective in the treatment of various indications and would be of great benefit in the public health sector. Accordingly, almost all the homoeopaths responding (96%) were convinced that the use of homoeopathy could reduce health care costs.

In contrast, a little under two-thirds (62%) of the directors of university medical departments completely reject payment of homoeopathic treatment by health insurance carriers, and a large majority (79%) of this occupational group was not prepared to pay privately for such treatment either. This unwillingness of directors of university medical departments to pay for homoeopathic treatment either via health insurance or privately, reflects their largely negative assessment of the value of such treatment.

An interesting observation was the fact that some two-thirds of the representatives of the health insurance carriers (64%) and politicians (69%) declared themselves willing to pay privately for such treatment. In contrast, the payment of homoeopathic treatment by health insurance carriers was favoured by only 50% and politicians 42%, respectively, of these two occupational groups. The willingness of these two groups to pay for homoeopathic treatment out of their own pockets rather than having it paid for by health insurance carriers, suggests that – in the light of a lack of convincing evaluative studies and the controversial discussions surrounding such treatment – their views reflect a strong sense of responsibility vis-à-vis the expenditure of public funds rather than their private convictions and beliefs.

The aim of the present epidemiological investigation was to define the socio-political and socio-economic status quo of homoeopathy as a complementary medical treatment, among decision-takers and service providers in the public health sector in five EU core countries. The data show that the assessments by supporters and opponents of homoeopathy of the parameters investigated are in some cases almost completely opposing. In particular homoeopaths and directors of university medical departments take up largely opposite positions with regard to the value of homoeopathy. Responses to this question appear to be highly dependent on the subjective experience of the respondents.

To date only a few high quality clinical scientific studies confirming the effectiveness of homoeopathy in selected indications have been carried out. An evaluation of the future sociopolitical and socioeconomic status of homoeopathy can be made only on the basis of more unequivocal data – which must be provided by relevant scientific research.

References

Aldridge, D. (1989) Europe looks at complementary medicine. *BMJ*, **299**, 1121–2.

Clinical Oncology Group (1987) New Zealand cancer patients and alternative medicine. *NZ Med. J.*, **100** (818), 110–13.

Eisenberg, D.M., Kessler, R.C., Foster, C., Norlock, F.E., Calkins, D.R. and Delbanco, T.L. (1993) Unconventional medicine in the United States. *N. Engl. J. Med.*, **328**, 246–52.

Ernst, E. (1995) Komplementärmedizin in der Jahresübersicht 1994. *Forsch. Komplementärmedizin*, **2**, 116–22.

Fisher, P. and Ward, A. (1994) Complementary medicine in Europe. *BMJ*, **309** (6947), 107–11.

Fisher, P. (1994) European initiatives and homoeopathy. *British Homoeopathic Journal*, **83**, 193–4.

Institut für Markt- und Werbeforschung Köln (1993) Repräsentativumfrage im Auftrag des Innungskrankenkassen-Bundesverbandes.

Klein, K.B. (1988) Controlled treatment trials in the irritable bowel syndrome: a critique. *Gastroenterology*, Jul, **95** (1), 232–41.

Kleijnen, J., Knipschild, P. and ter Riet, G. (1991) Clinical trials of homoeopathy. *BMJ*, **302**, 316–23.

Knipschild, P., Kleijnen, G. and ter Riet, G. (1990) Belief in the efficacy of alternative medicine among general practitioners in the Netherlands. *Soc. Sci. Med.*, **31**, 625–6.

L'Homéopathie en 1993. Lyons: Syndicat National de la Pharmacie Homéopathique 1993.

Linde, K., Clausius, N., Ramirez, G., Melchart, D., Eitel, F., Hedges, L.V. and Jonas, W.B. Are the Clinical Effects of Homoeopathy all Placebo Effects? A Meta-Analysis of Randomized, Placebo Controlled Trials. Submitted, not yet published, 1998.

Marshall, R.J., Gee, R., Israel, M., Neave, D., Edwards, F., Dumble, J., Wong, S., Chan, C., Patel, R., Poon, P. and Tam, G. (1990) The use of alternative therapies by Auckland general practitioners. *NZ Med. J.*, **103**, 213–15.

Matthiessen, P.F., Roßlenbroich, B. and Schmidt, S. (1992a) Unkonventionelle medizinische Richtungen. *Natur- und GanzheitsMedizin*, **5**, 7–15.

Matthiessen, P.F., Roßlenbroich, B. and Schmidt, S. (1992b) Unkonventionelle Medizinische Richtungen–Bestandsaufnahme zur Forschungssituation. Schriftenreihe zum Programm der Bundesregierung Forschung und Entwicklung im Dienste der Gesundheit. Bd 21. Wirtschaftsverlag NW, Bremerhaven, 1992.

Northcott, H.C. and Bachynsky, J.A. (1993) Concurrent utilization of chiropractic, prescription medicines, nonprescription medicines and alternative health care. *Soc. Sci. Med.*, **37**, 431–5.

Schneider, M., Biene-Dietrich, P., Gabanyi, M., Huber, M., Köse, A., Scholtes, L. and Sommer, J.H. (1993) Gesundheitssysteme im internationalen Vergleich. Augsburg, BASYS.

Schüppel, R. and Meinhold, M. (1994) Homöopathie – Ein Beitrag zur Kostendämpfung? *Der Kassenarzt*, **26**, 37–9.

Thomas, K.J., Westlake, L. and Williams, B.T. (1991) Use of non-orthodox and conventional health care in Great Britain. *BMJ*, **302**, 207–10.

Yates, P., Beadle, G., Clavarino, A., Najman, J.M., Thomson, D., Williams, G., Kenny, S., Roberts, B., Mason, B. and Schlect, D. (1993) Patients with terminal cancer who use alternative therapies: Their beliefs and practices. *Sociol. Health Illness*, **5**, 199–216.

Conclusions

Edzard Ernst and *Eckhart G. Hahn*

The controversies surrounding homoeopathy are as old as homoeopathy itself. As early as 1842 the arguments were wryly summarized by Oliver Wendel Holmes: '... when one man claims to have established these three independent truths (the three "axioms" that form the basis of homoeopathy), which are about as remote from each other as the discovery of the law of gravitation, the invention of printing, and that of the mariner's compass, unless the facts in their favour are overwhelming and unanimous, the question naturally arises, "is this man not deceiving himself, or trying to deceive others?"' (Holmes, 1989). Since then, the criticism has not ceased and only became less when homoeopathy was in decline. Today homoeopathy is popular again, and modern critics are keen to point out that homoeopathy has all the qualities of a sect (Jarvis, 1994) and represents 'a media-hyped superstition' (Meyer, 1996).

Two hundred years of such criticism, we believe, is quite enough. It has not proven to be productive and confuses doctors, scientists and patients alike. Therefore, this book is an attempt to critically review the evidence by bringing together experts who summarize what is known today.

The first section of the book relates to research methodology. All too often homoeopaths have tried to convince us that standard methods cannot be applied in their field. However, this argument simply does not hold water. The three chapters make clear that trial methodology in homoeopathy can be similar to that in mainstream medicine. It may (and often does) require thoughtful adaptation to meet the special requirements of homoeopathy. But certainly the wheel does not need to be re-invented. As in other fields of investigation the clinical trial is not the only way of acquiring knowledge, and the concluding chapter in this section deals with the important issue of other research methods applicable to homoeopathy. Such methods are not in competition with clinical trials; they are complementary in the true sense of the word.

The following section relates to provings, which form the very basis for homoeopathic prescribing. The underlying logic is explained and an informed critique of the evidence available to date is given. The reader is left with a feeling of uneasiness; this part of homoeopathy's fundament seems shaky indeed. At the same time it is becoming clear that research into provings could well be one of the most fruitful areas of investigation for homoeopaths. This section therefore can be viewed as an attempt to establish a firm basis for future, essential research into homoeopathic provings.

The central part of the book deals with the clinical aspects of homoeopathy. We analyse whether it is effective, efficacious and safe. A careful meta-analysis comes out in favour of homoeopathy. Yet, as with similar exercises, one needs to point out several caveats. The published trials are not all of high quality. Publication bias may have distorted the overall picture. And heterogeneity of the published data represents another serious problem. Frustratingly, the reader is therefore left without a firm YES or NO. The issue is complex and we need to consider placebo phenomena which are discussed in detail in the subsequent two chapters.

We often hear the somewhat naive opinion that, regardless whether homoeopathy is effective in a specific sense, at least it can do no harm. This issue too is more complex than it seems at first glance. Adverse reactions to homoeopathic remedies do occur but are probably rare. Then there is the confusing issue of 'homoeopathic aggravation'. Does this phenomenon really exist? Even homoeopaths are not entirely sure. And if it exists, don't we need to classify it as an adverse reaction? Finally there are indirect safety issues: even if homoeopathic remedies were entirely safe, not all homoeopaths are always safe.

The next section attempts to answer a question that has fascinated scientists for decades. Are highly diluted homoeopathic remedies in any way distinguishable from pure diluent? Some lines of evidence seem to indicate that this could indeed be the case. The critical reader, however, will remember the 'Benveniste affaire' (Maddox *et al.*, 1988) and will therefore rightly insist on independent replications of such results. We may or may not be convinced about the hypothesis apparently explaining the notion of 'memory of water', but theories and hypotheses must not be confused with scientific proof.

The final section represents an attempt to put homoeopathy into psycho-socio-economic context. Who uses homoeopathy and why? Does homoeopathy save money for either the individual or society? And why is there so little acceptance of homoeopathy? These are relevant questions at a time when the popularity of homoeopathy on the one hand and its implausibility and rejection by the 'establishment' on the other hand is a continuous puzzle to many.

The book spans the entire spectrum from qualitative to quantitative research, from laboratory to clinical investigation, from medical to sociological questions. By no means will it settle the debate about homoeopathy, but it will most certainly inform this debate by providing the 'state of the art' and up-to-date, balanced analysis. An overall conclusion seems to emerge: Homoeopathy can be researched largely by conventional methods. Perhaps surprisingly, the most fundamental questions in homoeopathy are not yet answered conclusively – but there seems to be light at the end of the tunnel.

References

Holmes, O.W. (1989) *Homoeopathy and its kindred delusions*. First published 1842, republished in D. Stalker, C. Glymour *Examining holistic medicine*. Buffalo, NY: Prometheus Books.

Jarvis, W. (1994) Homeopathy, a position statement by the national council against health fraud. *Skeptic*, **3**, 50–7.

Maddox, J., Randi, J., Stewart, W.W. (1988) 'High dilution' experiments a delusion. *Nature*, **333**, 287–90.

Meyer, F.P. (1996) Vorlesungen über Homöopathie. Fischer: Jena.

Index

Note: page references in *italics* indicate tables or figures; there may also be relevant text on these pages